Balance Restored

A Comprehensive Guide to Women's Hormone Health

Olivia Rivers

© **Copyright 2023 - All rights reserved.**

The content contained within this book may not be reproduced, duplicated, or transmitted without direct written permission from the author or the publisher.

Under no circumstances will any blame or legal responsibility be held against the publisher, or author, for any damages, reparation, or monetary loss due to the information contained within this book, either directly or indirectly.

Legal Notice:

This book is copyright protected. It is only for personal use. You cannot amend, distribute, sell, use, quote or paraphrase any part, or the content within this book, without the consent of the author or publisher.

Disclaimer Notice:

Please note the information contained within this document is for educational and entertainment purposes only. All effort has been executed to present accurate, up to date, reliable, complete information. No warranties of any kind are declared or implied. Readers acknowledge that the author is not engaged in the rendering of legal, financial, medical, or professional advice. The content within this book has been derived from various sources. Please consult a licensed professional before attempting any techniques outlined in this book.

By reading this document, the reader agrees that under no circumstances is the author responsible for any losses, direct or indirect, that are incurred as a result of the use of the information contained within this document, including, but not limited to, errors, omissions, or inaccuracies.

An Exclusive Gift Awaits You!

Unlock Your Hormone-Supporting Recipe Guide Now!

As you delve into the empowering pages of "Balance Restored," we're delighted to offer you an exclusive companion – "Balanced Bites." This invaluable eBook is a tribute to your journey of reclaiming hormonal harmony and vitality.

Enclosed within, you'll discover a treasure trove of wisdom – a succinct exploration of crucial nutrients that play pivotal roles in nurturing hormone health, your essential shopping list for fostering hormonal balance, and a delectable array of hormone-balancing recipes for breakfast, lunch, dinner, snacks, and desserts. Each recipe is accompanied by its related nutritional information, providing you with the tools to nourish and revitalize your well-being.

To access your special gift, simply scan the QR code below and follow the prompts.

Embrace this opportunity to nourish your body, balance your hormones, and embark on a remarkable journey toward holistic well-being.

Table of Contents

INTRODUCTION 1

CHAPTER 1: UNDERSTANDING HORMONES 5

WHAT IS A HORMONE? 6
WHAT DO HORMONES DO? 6
   Growth Hormone (Human Growth Hormone) 7
   Norepinephrine (Noradrenaline) 8
   Sex Hormones 9
   Thyroid Hormones 9
   Insulin and Glucagon 10
   Oxytocin 11
THE KEY HORMONES THAT AFFECT WOMEN'S HEALTH 11
   Estrogen 12
   Progesterone 12
   Luteinizing Hormone (LH) 13
   Follicle Stimulating Hormone (FSH) 14
   Testosterone 14
HOW HORMONES REACT WITH EACH OTHER 15
   Conclusion 16

CHAPTER 2: HORMONAL LIFE STAGES FOR WOMEN 19

FEMALE PUBERTY 20
THE REPRODUCTIVE YEARS 21
   The Menstrual Cycle 21
   Perimenopause 22
   Menopause 23
   Common Conditions in the Reproductive Years 23
   Dysmenorrhea 25
   Amenorrhea 26
OTHER CONSIDERATIONS 26
   Conclusion 27

CHAPTER 3: SIGNS AND SYMPTOMS OF HORMONAL IMBALANCE 29

THE PROBLEM OF SELF-DIAGNOSIS 30

THE WIDE-RANGING SIGNS AND SYMPTOMS OF HORMONAL IMBALANCES......... 31
   How Hormones Affect the Body 32
   How to Identify Hormonal Imbalances 35
A HOLISTIC APPROACH 36
   Start Making Changes 37
   Managing Your Hormone Health More Effectively....................... 38
   Conclusion 40

CHAPTER 4: CAUSES OF HORMONAL IMBALANCES............................ 43

GENETIC CONDITIONS 43
   What Is a Hereditary Disease?.. 44
   What to Do if a Disease Runs in Your Family 45
   Type 2 Diabetes 46
   Polycystic Ovary Syndrome... 47
   Hashimoto's Disease.. 48
LIFESTYLE FACTORS: DIET, EXERCISE, STRESS, AND SLEEP 50
   Diet 50
   Exercise 51
   Sleep 53
ENVIRONMENTAL FACTORS 54
   Conclusion 55

CHAPTER 5: EFFECTS OF HORMONAL IMBALANCES 57

   Impact on Physical Health 57
   Impacts on Mental and Emotional Health..................................... 58
   Well-Being and Quality of Life 59
   Early Detection and Mitigation... 60
CONCLUSION 62

CHAPTER 6: HORMONES AND NUTRITION 63

THE NUTRITIONAL HORMONES 63
   Ghrelin 63
   Leptin... 64
   Gastrointestinal Hormones... 64
   Insulin 64
   Glucagon 65
THE PROBLEM OF EXTREME DIETING... 65
NUTRIENTS AND HOW THEY AFFECT YOUR HORMONES.............................. 67
   Micronutrients 67
   Overnutrition 68
   Malnutrition 69

Conclusion *70*

CHAPTER 7: LIFESTYLE MANAGEMENT FOR HORMONE HEALTH **71**

Stress *71*
DIFFERENT TYPES OF STRESS 74
Stress Management: Tips, Tricks, and Techniques *76*
CULTIVATING A HEALTHY ENVIRONMENT 77
Maintaining a Healthy Sleep Schedule *78*
A Balanced Diet *79*
Maintaining Movement *81*
Regular Exercise: Strength and Cardio *83*
Stretching and Strengthening: Yoga and Pilates *84*
CONCLUSION 85

CHAPTER 8: NATURAL REMEDIES AND SUPPLEMENTS FOR HORMONAL HEALTH **87**

Supplements: The Science *88*
ADAPTOGENS 89
Ashwagandha *90*
Aloe Vera *91*
Rhodiola *91*
Suggested Supplements List *92*
THE DANGERS OF SUPPLEMENTS 93
CONCLUSION 95

CHAPTER 9: MEDICAL INTERVENTIONS **97**

WHAT MEDICAL INTERVENTIONS ARE AVAILABLE? 98
HOW TO ADVOCATE FOR YOURSELF 101
Be Smart About Your Research *102*
Write Down What You Want to Say *102*
Challenge, Challenge, Challenge *103*
Conclusion *103*

CHAPTER 10: COMMUNICATING HORMONAL HEALTH CONCERNS .. **105**

THE CONVERSATION 106
Documenting Your Symptoms *106*
WHAT TO DO 108
Menopause and Perimenopause *109*
Hormone Replacement Therapy *109*
Polycystic Ovary Syndrome (PCOS) *110*
Take Your Time *111*

    Seek a Second Opinion *112*
    CONCLUSION 112

CHAPTER 11: PREVENTATIVE MEASURES AND LONG-TERM MAINTENANCE 115

    LIFESTYLE TWEAKS 115
        Building Habits *116*
        Supplements *116*
        Physical Activity *117*
        Change Your Environment *118*
    STRESS MANAGEMENT STRATEGIES 120
    HEALTH SCREENINGS: A REMINDER 122
    CONCLUSION 123

CHAPTER 12: RESOURCES AND COMMUNITIES 125

    ONLINE RESOURCES 125
        Websites and Forums *125*
        Blogs and Articles *126*
        Podcasts *126*
    BOOKS 127

CONCLUSION 129

REFERENCES 135

Introduction

Hormone health is at the core of women's health, which is why balancing hormones is such an important topic. A woman's body is capable of achieving homeostasis—a state of balance—by producing hormones that govern a wide variety of functions. Your body uses hormones for everything from your estrogen and progesterone levels during your menstrual cycle to the enzymes in your gut that assist with digestion. The body is capable of taking care of itself, but as we age and contend with day-to-day life, it needs a lot of help from us. Unfortunately, when these hormones become unbalanced, it can cause various health problems.

These health problems range from slight discomfort during premenstrual syndrome (PMS) all the way to severe bouts of depression during menopause. To be a woman navigating her own health is to be constantly aware that her health is affected by her hormonal balance and other factors. According to a 2023 report by Northwell Health, up to 80% of women suffer from hormonal imbalances and 70% are unaware that some conditions can be caused by hormonal imbalances (Travers, 2023). Conditions, such as polycystic ovary syndrome (PCOS) and endometriosis (where tissue similar to the uterine lining grows outside of the uterus), have hormonal causes.

And then we get into a woman's key hormonal life stages: puberty, menstruation, perimenopause, and menopause.

Hormones are a critical part of a woman's health. At the time of writing this book, over 50 hormones have been identified. In addition to estrogen and progesterone, hormones such as insulin, ghrelin, human growth hormone, adrenaline, and countless others all work together to keep the body in a state of balance, and internal and external factors can easily knock them out of balance. The stress cycle, for example, is an internal process that influences the release of cortisol and adrenaline. It's important to remember that not all stress is bad; if anything, it's necessary for certain functions to take place. External factors, such as exercise, cause the stress cycle to take place. This influences the release of human growth hormone and some androgens (such as testosterone), which leads to muscle growth and repair, resulting in increased muscle mass and bone density.

Our knowledge of women's health is expansive yet limited in many ways. For example, we know that conditions such as endometriosis exist, but the process of receiving a diagnosis is long and costly. For decades—centuries even—women's issues have been looked down upon and reduced to "hormonal issues" or "*that* time of the month." Hippocrates coined the term "hysteria" to describe a condition where a woman's uterus detaches itself and floats around the body, causing a variety of female illnesses. However, we now use the term "hysteria" to refer to exaggerated or uncontrollable excitement, or the word "hysterical" describes something extremely funny.

Something we need to factor in is that we live in the digital age. While the digital age has improved connection and communication, linking us to infinite information, it has also linked us to an onslaught of misinformation. All over the world, women are being encouraged to pursue dangerous practices in the name of hormone health, and quick warning: It's about to get gross. I recently saw a reel on Instagram where a woman was encouraging her viewers to drink their own urine as part of her practice. I should not need to remind you that urine is a *waste product* and that drinking it can have disastrous effects on your physical health. If you come across a reel, TikTok, or other social media content similar to this, I would encourage you to press the block button because misinformation can be very detrimental and dangerous.

I will admit, I have been a victim of misinformation. Like most women, I was carrying a few extra pounds at the end of the pandemic, and I wanted them gone as soon as possible. While I was going to the gym and eating a balanced diet, the pounds weren't shifting as much as I wanted them to. In the end, I started looking up "fast ways to lose weight and keep it off." Fat loss does not work like that. Through my own research, I have come to learn that hormones play a subtle role in fat loss.

At the time, I didn't realize that exercise played a role in hormone regulation. When I first started exercising, I just knew that I felt good. Then, I signed up for a program that required me to exercise six days a week and eat three meals a day, supplemented with protein shakes. This went on for about eight weeks before I started feeling dizzy, tired, and lethargic. When I went to the doctor to get a blood panel, it came back that my blood sugar was low, which meant that my insulin levels were low. I dropped the protocol and went back to my old routine. At my next appointment, my insulin levels had gone back to normal.

Misinformation preys on vulnerable women who want nothing more than to improve their health. Instead of participating in dangerous practices, women should be learning about what their hormones actually are and what they do. Moreover, women should be focusing on what they can do, here and now, to bring balance to their hormones *safely*. That's the key: safety.

This book is here to set the record straight. Over the course of the next few chapters, we are going to look at the different hormones present in a woman's body, navigate what they do, and how we can best look after this magnificent biological machine that keeps us going. I hope that, by the end of this book, you will understand one thing: Your body is incredible, but it needs a little help every now and then, and it is your prerogative to look after your body to the best of your ability.

Chapter 1:

Understanding Hormones

Before we get into how to balance our hormones, we need to first understand what hormones are, their function in the body, and which hormones specifically affect women's health. For the most part, this is going to be a crash course or a reminder of all the things we learned in science class many years ago. A lot of new information has come out in recent years, including research proving how important hormone balance is for women.

Though they may not seem so important at first, hormones can profoundly affect our body's growth and development, metabolism, sexual function, reproduction, mood, and more. An imbalance, whether in deficiency or excess, can significantly impact a woman's health.

Later on, we'll explore how hormones affect women in later stages of life. Hormones shift on a daily and lifetime basis. The hormone levels you have now are probably not the same as the levels they were at last year! It's perfectly natural for hormonal balance to shift over time, and we need to be prepared for when that happens. As we go further into the complex nature of hormones, we are going to understand just how vital it is to keep them balanced.

Later, we will look at the importance of hormone balance, the signs and symptoms, causes, and how we might be able to remedy the imbalance. This includes managing hormone balance through diet, lifestyle changes, and potentially through medical intervention.

What Is a Hormone?

Hormones are powerful chemical messengers in the body, produced by the endocrine glands. They travel in our bloodstream to tissues and organs, regulating our bodily functions. Important hormones that significantly affect women's health, such as estrogen, progesterone, follicle-stimulating hormone (FSH), luteinizing hormone (LH), thyroid hormones, cortisol, and insulin, will be discussed extensively.

The adrenal glands, which are found on top of your kidneys, are responsible for producing adrenaline and cortisol. The pituitary gland is responsible for producing human growth hormone, also known as growth hormone.

To date, 50 hormones have been identified in the body, and all of them are very important. The balance of each is vital to the body's ability to keep itself alive. Although we are not going to look at all 50 hormones, we are going to look at the hormones that are the most important to women's health.

What Do Hormones Do?

Hormones are a key component in many physiological changes that occur in the body. These include appetite, puberty, growth, and fertility. Some hormones are required more often than others, while others are needed in great quantities during specific times of life, only to be needed in smaller quantities later.

Some hormones are known as steroid hormones, which are steroids that behave in a similar way to a hormone. Androgens, progestogens, and estrogens are all classified as steroid hormones. Yes, this means that your sex hormones, which we will cover in this section, are classed as steroids. The word "steroids" has a negative connotation because of their illicit use in the world of competitive sports.

However, the steroids used in competitive sports are actually man-made versions of naturally occurring hormones. These steroids, however, have many other applications, aside from giving athletes an unfair advantage. For example, women who need supplemental estrogen during and after menopause will receive it. The estrogen they are taking is a man-made version of estrogen.

I assure you that there is nothing illicit about your hormones being steroids. They are naturally occurring, and the body produces them in the quantities it needs, assuming that there are no issues with your hormonal balance.

Growth Hormone (Human Growth Hormone)

Growth hormone—also referred to as human growth hormone (HGH) and by its chemical name, somatotropin—is the driving factor that stimulates growth, cell reproduction, and cell regeneration. It can be found in both humans and animals, although in this context we are interested in its human form. During puberty, your pituitary gland secretes a massive amount of HGH to stimulate a growth spurt and the development of your reproductive system.

Your body is not done with human growth hormone when puberty has finished. In fact, your body continues to secrete it during several phases of life. Levels of it even fluctuate during daily life. The best example I can give is that the recovery period after intense exercise involves human growth hormone. Muscle fibers break down, and human growth hormone helps them repair and grow stronger, in both size and shape. Growth hormone can be given as a supplement in children who are delayed in puberty.

Stress Hormones

Adrenaline and Cortisol

Adrenaline plays an important role in regulating your heartbeat and helping you breathe more efficiently. When we get stressed or experience a sudden burst of fear, our heart rate speeds up, and we begin to hyperventilate. This is a result of increased adrenaline in the bloodstream. Without it, we would not have a functional fight-or-flight response. During an allergic reaction, you might be given a shot of adrenaline, referred to as epinephrine.

Cortisol has multiple roles in the body, including supporting the immune system and regulating the metabolism. It is a steroid hormone. If you are experiencing prolonged periods of stress, you might have a bit too much cortisol in your system. You may notice weight gain (especially in the face and abdomen), high blood pressure, and even muscle weakness. While cortisol is an important hormone, it's possible to have too much of a good thing.

Norepinephrine (Noradrenaline)

Norepinephrine, also called noradrenaline, is a fascinating hormone because it is both a hormone and a neurotransmitter. Norepinephrine is produced in the adrenal glands. Its function is to fuel the fight-or-flight response. Its purpose is to transmit signals across the body's nerve endings. It increases your sense of alertness, attention to detail, as well as your arousal. You might notice a slight constriction of your blood vessels, but this is nothing to worry about (unless you have high blood pressure). This is simply norepinephrine doing its job to maintain your blood pressure when you are stressed.

Sex Hormones

Sex hormones are categorized by their effects on sexual desire, reproduction, and sexual characteristics. In women, the main sex hormones are estrogen and progesterone. In men, it's testosterone.

Estrogen can be broken down by the body into 2-hydroxyestrone and 16-hydroxyestrone, each of which has a different function. The body uses 2-hydroxyestrone to block stronger estrogen hormones and may inhibit cancer growth. 16-hydroxyestrone promotes bone density. Estradiol is another type of estrogen, which can be given orally to help reduce the symptoms of menopause.

Testosterone can be converted into dihydrotestosterone, which stimulates body hair growth and sexual organ function, among other things.

Thyroid Hormones

Feel along the base of your neck, around the top of your collarbone. It's around here that you will find your thyroid gland. If you were to look at it on a diagram, it's the gland shaped like a butterfly. Your thyroid gland produces triiodothyronine and thyroxine, which you might see referred to as T3 and T4, respectively. These two hormones play very important roles in the body, including the regulation of weight, energy levels throughout the day, blood pressure, heart rate, thermogenesis (body temperature), and the health of your skin, hair, and nails. Your metabolism, which is the sum of all chemical processes occurring in the body is also maintained by

T3 and T4. The thyroid is susceptible to cancer, although the precise cause of this is unknown. According to the American Thyroid Association, "Thyroid cancer has always been diagnosed more commonly in women than in men" (Sulanc, 2021).

Parathyroid hormone is another important thyroid hormone to be aware of. The parathyroids can be found either side of the thyroid, and each one is quite small, no bigger than a pea. They secrete parathyroid hormones that regulate calcium concentration and its effects throughout the bones, kidneys, and intestines.

Insulin and Glucagon

Insulin is a hormone that is produced by the pancreas. It is released in response to the presence of glucose. Although it has many functions in the human body, its primary purpose is to convert glucose from the food we eat into glycogen. Sometimes glycogen can be stored in the muscles, so you might hear it referred to as "muscle glycogen." Another of insulin's roles is to regulate blood sugar. When blood sugar gets too high (known as hyperglycemia, high glucose presence in the blood), insulin is released to bring the levels down by metabolizing the excess glucose.

A counterpart to insulin, a very important one too, is glucagon. Glucagon also regulates blood sugar levels. When blood sugar is too low (known as hypoglycemia, low glucose presence in blood) the pancreas releases glucagon to stimulate the production of glucose and the release of glycogen from the liver. This is called glycogenolysis, a process that brings glucose levels back to normal.

Oxytocin

Another hormone you will find in your pituitary gland is oxytocin. Oxytocin is usually called the "bonding" hormone for its role in social bonding. However, it has other functions as it is a behavioral hormone. In women, oxytocin is released in several circumstances, including childbirth, while breastfeeding, and in response to touch. Oxytocin is created by the hypothalamus and stored by the pituitary gland.

Oxytocin is also nicknamed the "love hormone." This is because it's released when we are with our romantic or sexual partner or when we're around those we love. Oxytocin regulates emotional responses, allowing us to build relationships. For example, if your best friend smiles at you, you will get a short hit of oxytocin. If you are holding hands with your partner, you will get a hit of oxytocin. If you are having dinner with friends and laughing about a shared experience, you will get a hit of oxytocin. This hormone is important because it helps cultivate empathy, trust, and bonding.

The Key Hormones That Affect Women's Health

Now that we've covered some of the general hormones, let's look at the major hormones that affect women's health. Often, women's issues are reduced to the state of hormones, and while this might be true in some cases, in others it's blatantly false. We all have hormonal fluctuations that affect our moods but what is less understood is how hormones affect women's health to begin with. Let's take a look at the major hormones that affect your health as a woman, where they are secreted from, and the role they play in your body.

Estrogen

Estrogen is responsible for the female reproductive system, its growth and development, and its physiology. In females, it is produced in the ovaries. Technically, "estrogen" is an umbrella term given to a group of three hormones: estradiol, estrone, and estriol. All three are important, but the major hormone here is estradiol. Estradiol's main function is to mature and release the egg during ovulation, while estrone helps with the development of the reproductive system and estriol helps the uterus stay healthy.

Symptoms of estrogen deficiency:

- Dry skin
- Tender breasts
- Vaginal atrophy
- Vaginal dryness
- Hot flashes
- Night sweats

Progesterone

During the early stages of your period, the lining of the uterus (the endometrium) thickens, preparing for a fertilized egg. Progesterone is the hormone responsible for this thickening of the endometrium. If there is no fertilized egg, the endometrium breaks up and sheds, creating your period. In the event implantation occurs, progesterone secretion increases to support pregnancy.

Symptoms of progesterone deficiency:

- Irregular periods
- Fertility issues
- Difficulty sleeping
- Bloating
- Weight gain
- Changes in mood

Luteinizing Hormone (LH)

Luteinizing hormone (LH) is the hormone that causes ovulation. It is secreted by the pituitary gland and governs sexual development, sexual functioning, and the regulation of the menstrual cycle.

Symptoms of luteinizing hormone (LH) deficiency:

- Difficulty making breast milk (if lactating)
- Loss of pubic hair
- Irritability and other changes in mood
- Lethargy, tiredness, and fatigue

Follicle Stimulating Hormone (FSH)

Follicle-stimulating hormone (FSH) is another hormone that regulates the menstrual cycle by stimulating the growth of ova (eggs). Throughout the menstrual cycle, follicle-stimulating hormone levels can fluctuate, the highest levels being just before the ovary releases the egg.

Symptoms of follicle-stimulating hormone (FSH) deficiency:

- Difficulty getting pregnant
- Irregular periods
- Lack of ability to lactate
- Loss of libido

Testosterone

Although it is considered an androgen or a "male hormone," women need testosterone. While women don't have nearly as much testosterone as men, it still plays a vital function in women's health. In fact, estrogen and testosterone work together to maintain and grow reproductive tissues and develop bone density.

Symptoms of testosterone deficiency:

- Fatigue
- Muscle loss
- Reduced libido

- Weight gain

How Hormones React with Each Other

In addition to the above hormones, there are a variety of other hormones that affect the human body. Hormones are just a small part of your body, and they work together (sometimes against each other), to keep your body running at an optimal level. For example, when we exercise, adrenaline and cortisol are released to prevent us from feeling pain. Exercise, especially intense exercise like weight lifting, can cause microtears in the muscles. As you can imagine, this is intense and would be very painful, if we didn't have adrenaline and cortisol blocking the pain.

When the hormones work together, they do it for the benefit of our survival. Melatonin is released when we get tired, so we yawn, feel drowsy, and fall asleep. Melatonin also prevents the secretion of estradiol, which can cause decreased fertility in women. Some scholars suggest that melatonin could be a viable treatment for infertility in women, although studies in this area are ongoing (Starr, 2011).

Ghrelin is also known as "the hunger hormone." When the stomach is empty, ghrelin is released. It then acts on the hypothalamus in the brain to signal that it's time to eat. That's when you start hearing your stomach rumbling and feeling its emptiness. Ghrelin works with another hormone, leptin, which is secreted when you're full. Leptin has also been reported to increase levels of luteinizing hormone (Gao and Horvath, 2008).

Insulin is secreted in response to glucose. When glucose is present in the blood, insulin is released to convert it into glycogen so that it can be stored in the muscles. When glucose levels are low, insulin is not secreted.

Insulin and progesterone may have a unique relationship. Some evidence indicates that progesterone blocks insulin receptors in the body, which can cause you to feel sluggish, lethargic, and maybe even a little bit hungry (Yeung et al., 2010). More recent studies have found that progesterone might also cause gluconeogenesis, which is the process of the body converting dietary fat to glucose (Lee et al., 2020).

Progesterone causes elevated levels of glucose in the blood, also known as high blood sugar levels. This might explain why we feel a little more energetic during certain phases of the menstrual cycle. On the other hand, estrogen causes a decrease in blood sugar, which can cause lethargy and tiredness during the early stage of the menstrual cycle.

Another hormone that reacts with progesterone is adrenaline. Adrenaline, as we have established, is one of the key stress hormones that is secreted during times of stress. Progesterone increases in response to stress, although it is not clear why (Herrera et al., 2016). On the topic of stress hormones, high levels of cortisol can block the secretion of estrogen and progesterone. Have you ever been so stressed that your period was late? Well, that's why. Because your levels of cortisol were so high, in order to relieve this stress, your body limited the production of estrogen and progesterone.

Conclusion

Hormones are vital chemical messengers produced by our endocrine system; they govern many aspects of our bodies, such as growth, metabolism, sexual function, and reproduction.

Estrogen, progesterone, follicle-stimulating hormone (FSH), luteinizing hormone (LH), thyroid hormones, cortisol, and insulin. These hormones work together to maintain homeostasis in the body and keep you healthy. While these hormones work together, they can also work against each other. For example, cortisol can block the production of estrogen, which can delay the menstrual cycle and prevent a period from occurring. It is the body's way of reducing stress.

Finally, an imbalance of hormones, either too much or too little, can lead to serious health concerns. Endometriosis occurs when tissue like the uterine lining grows outside of the uterus. Endometriosis is a serious condition that can cause severe, crippling pelvic pain and reduce fertility. It can occur at any time—when you have your first period or later in life—and it can last all the way until menopause. In extreme cases, endometriosis can be fatal. We will look at endometriosis and other conditions later on.

Now that we have a firm foundation on these female hormones, let's move on and explore the different hormone cycles a woman will go through throughout her life.

Chapter 2:

Hormonal Life Stages for Women

Hormones move in cycles. They fluctuate, just like life. At times, your period can be the most consistent cycle you've ever experienced, and you can track it. But hormones rise and fall at points in life including pregnancy, postpartum (the period of time after giving birth), perimenopause ("around menopause," the time when your body naturally transitions toward menopause), and menopause (the time in a woman's life when her fertility ceases).

It's unfortunate that so much of women's health or stress is dismissed as "hormonal issues." Understanding these "hormonal issues" is the very key to our health! Hormones can, and do, affect our emotional, physical, and mental health. When the body experiences low levels of thyroid hormones, this can result in a slow metabolism, which can lead to weight gain, and conditions like hypothyroidism (a condition where the thyroid is underactive).

Hormonal imbalances can cause a variety of issues. Polycystic ovary syndrome (PCOS) causes cysts to grow on the ovaries and results in difficulty getting pregnant, a loss of weight, and an irregular menstrual cycle. In addition to being caused by hormonal imbalances, polycystic ovary syndrome (PCOS) can cause them as well. It is also known that PCOS can cause high levels of estrogen and low levels of progesterone. At the time of writing this book, there is no known cause of PCOS.

In this chapter, we are going to explore how hormones shift and change over the course of a woman's life, beginning in girlhood and adolescence through to menopause and beyond.

Female Puberty

Let's begin with the first significant hormonal transition: puberty. Puberty begins between the ages of 8 and 13, and it lasts well into the teenage years. By the time a girl is 18, she will stop growing; although in some cases, girls may stop growing a little later. In general, girls and children assigned female at birth will reach their adult height before puberty ends. The roles of estrogen, progesterone, follicle-stimulating hormone (FSH), and luteinizing hormone (LH) come into play during puberty, leading to the onset of menstruation in children assigned female at birth, and the development of secondary sexual characteristics.

Let's start with the physical changes. The earliest hormonal changes lead to one of the first physical changes: breast development. Breast buds form under the nipples. They are usually firm and tender. Over the next year or two, they will grow larger. Pubic hair also begins to grow and is typically dark, coarse, and curly. It grows on the vulva, which is the area around the vagina.

As for the internal hormonal changes, egg stimulation begins. Estrogen begins to be secreted, triggering the development and release of ova (eggs). Progesterone begins to thicken the lining of the uterus in preparation for menarche, your first period. Other hormonal changes include a rapid secretion of human growth hormone (HGH) which results in a growth spurt, as well as the growth of body hair, the development of body odor, and acne.

The Reproductive Years

After puberty comes one of the longest periods of hormonal fluctuations in a woman's life: the reproductive years. These hormonal fluctuations cause periods, which exist for the purpose of getting pregnant.

The Menstrual Cycle

The menstrual cycle has four phases: menstruation, the follicular phase, ovulation, and the luteal phase.

The best-known phase is menstruation, which is often referred to as your period. This occurs when the lining of the uterus sheds and flows from the vagina along with some blood and mucus. You can expect your period to last from three days up to a week, depending on the nature of the blood. Options such as tampons, sanitary pads, menstrual cups, and special period underwear are available to control the flow of blood.

On the first day of your period, you are in the follicular phase, and it can last for up to two weeks. This occurs when follicle-stimulating hormone (FSH) is released to stimulate the follicles that cover the top of the ovary. Around the 10-day mark of the cycle, one of the follicles will develop into an egg, and the lining of your uterus will thicken to prepare for implantation.

The follicle matures into an egg and is then released. The egg travels along the fallopian tube, heading toward the uterus, where it waits to be fertilized. Ovulation can last up to 32 hours and occurs about two weeks before your period is due to start. During this time, it's possible to get pregnant. Fertilization can occur from five days before ovulation to the day of ovulation, although you are most fertile in the three days before it occurs. Once released from the ovary, an ovum can last for up to 24 hours before being passed.

Once ovulation is finished, the corpus luteum (cells in the ovary) releases a little estrogen and some progesterone to thicken the uterus. This prepares the uterus for pregnancy. In the event of pregnancy, the corpus luteum will continue to release progesterone to maintain the uterine lining. If there is no pregnancy, progesterone levels drop as the corpus luteum dies, and the uterine lining sheds.

Perimenopause

Perimenopause is the transition to menopause. It literally means "around menopause" because it happens around the time your menstrual cycle stops, which signals that the reproductive years have come to an end. You might also hear perimenopause referred to as "the menopausal transition." They both mean the same thing.

No two women experience perimenopause the same way, but there are a few general signs and symptoms to look out for. During perimenopause, ovulation becomes erratic. You might have a slightly longer period than normal one month, only to have no period the next month. This happens because your ovaries gradually stop working. They stop producing the hormones required for reproduction.

Other signs to look out for include hot flashes, a disrupted sleep pattern, irritability, and vaginal dryness. Perimenopause usually starts in your early 40s and can vary in length. While some women might be in perimenopause for a few years, others might only experience it for a few months. No two women will have the exact same experience, but perimenopause does signal the onset of menopause.

Menopause

Menopause is a natural part of aging that occurs at the end of a woman's reproductive years. It happens between the ages of 45 and 55 when the ovaries finally stop producing estrogen, which is required to release an egg every month for menstruation. While it is a natural part of aging, some women who go through cancer treatments, specifically chemotherapy or radiotherapy, might experience early menopause. A woman who has had a full or partial hysterectomy might experience symptoms of menopause.

Symptoms to look out for include hot flashes, vaginal dryness, low mood, irritability, disrupted sleeping patterns, and night sweats. Treatment options are available, although not all women need them. Hormone replacement therapy to support bone density and mental health is usually offered, as well as cognitive behavioral therapy to support mental health during menopause. Some women opt for herbal treatments such as evening primrose oil and ginseng, although there is little evidence to support their efficacy.

Common Conditions in the Reproductive Years

Polycystic Ovary Syndrome

Polycystic ovary syndrome is a condition that affects 8–13% of women globally (*Polycystic Ovary Syndrome,* 2023). PCOS affects how the ovaries function and can cause irregular, heavy, and painful periods. As the name implies, polycystic ovary syndrome causes cysts to develop on the ovaries that disrupt the production and secretion of estrogen, leading to irregular ovulation and irregular periods.

Other symptoms to look out for include the growth of facial hair, difficulty getting pregnant, and difficulty losing weight. At present, it is not known exactly what causes polycystic ovary syndrome, although it is thought to be hormonal in nature. There are treatments available that target the symptoms rather than the cause. If you suffer from polycystic ovary syndrome, these treatments include fertility treatments, hormone replacement therapy, and medications that inhibit the growth of facial hair.

Premenstrual Syndrome

All women will experience premenstrual syndrome at some point in their life. It's an umbrella term referring to the symptoms women experience before a period occurs. You might get these symptoms the week before your period starts, the day before, or they might last all cycle long. It is not known exactly what causes premenstrual syndrome, but it is thought to be linked to the natural fluctuations of hormones during the menstrual cycle.

Symptoms of premenstrual syndrome can vary wildly. Where one woman might experience severe abdominal cramping, another might experience tiredness. Other symptoms include skin breakouts, headaches, mood swings, and mineral deficiencies such as iron deficiency anemia. Treatment options are widely available and include over-the-counter pain medications, hormone therapy in extreme cases, and plenty of bed rest.

Premenstrual Dysphoric Disorder

Premenstrual dysphoric disorder (PMDD) is like premenstrual syndrome (PMS) on steroids. It can be brutal. Where premenstrual syndrome (PMS) will make you feel weepy, a bit tired, and a little hungry, premenstrual dysphoric disorder (PMDD) is far more serious. Symptoms include severe irritability, extreme menstrual pain, lethargy, fatigue, depression, and crippling anxiety in the days leading up to your period. If premenstrual syndrome (PMS) makes you feel a bit sad during your period, premenstrual dysphoric disorder (PMDD) can wreck your mental health. A 2021 review found that women who suffer from PMDD are "almost seven times at higher risk of suicide attempt and almost four times as likely to exhibit suicidal ideation" (Prasad et al., 2021).

There aren't many treatment options for PMDD as it is treated in a similar way to PMS. Painkillers are often prescribed by healthcare providers and yoga and stretching are recommended to relieve tension in the lower back. Herbal teas are also recommended, and caffeine intake is suggested to be reduced. In some cases, women with premenstrual dysphoric disorder (PMDD) might be prescribed supplemental iron, B12, and zinc, among other vitamins and minerals, to reduce the risk of anemia during menstruation.

Dysmenorrhea

Dysmenorrhea is the name given to painful periods. Little is known about this, although it is suspected that hormonal changes might prompt the uterus to squeeze harder than necessary to shed its lining. Options for treatment include contraceptive pills and painkillers.

Amenorrhea

Amenorrhea is the absence of the menstrual period. This is completely normal in some cases, such as pregnancy, lactation, pre-puberty, and post-menopause. In other cases, such as during the reproductive years, this is considered to be abnormal. Many things can cause amenorrhea, including high and low body weight and excessive exercise.

Other Considerations

Before we move on, there are a few other considerations we should address. In particular, we should address how hormonal fluctuations and imbalances affect cardiovascular and bone health.

We touched briefly on cortisol imbalance in the previous chapter. A high concentration of this hormone can severely impact bone health. If left for too long, it can result in osteoporosis. It does this by affecting bone turnover, also called bone metabolism or bone remodeling. Bone turnover is a lifelong process that controls the shaping, reshaping, and replacement of the skeleton. This process also controls the replacement and healing of bones following breakages, fractures, and smaller damage or micro-damage, which may occur during daily activities.

Cortisol greatly affects this process by affecting the reabsorption of calcium through the renal system (kidneys). During perimenopause and menopause, cortisol can inhibit reproductive hormones.

Conclusion

Hormones undergo significant changes through different stages in a woman's life: puberty, reproductive years, pregnancy and postpartum, perimenopause, and menopause. Hormonal imbalances at any life stage can cause several health-related issues ranging from menstrual irregularities, such as PCOS, to emotional disturbances like postpartum depression and menopausal symptoms. Understanding these hormonal transitions can help women better navigate their health throughout these stages.

Hormonal shifts are normal. For women, these shifts are often misunderstood, and that misunderstanding leads to misinformation. Now that we understand how our hormones affect us during puberty, the reproductive years, perimenopause, and menopause, we are in a better position to take action. Hormonal imbalances can lead to significant changes in emotional, physical, and mental health. Without this vital understanding, we are left directionless in how we can act. In the next chapter, we are going to look at the signs and symptoms of hormonal imbalance.

Chapter 3:

Signs and Symptoms of Hormonal Imbalance

Hormonal imbalances can have many different signs and symptoms, indicating issues, and some will be more obvious than others. Varied hormones have distinct roles; thus, imbalances will present different symptoms. For instance, imbalances in sex hormones can result in symptoms such as infertility, irregular periods, or low sex drive. Alternatively, insulin imbalances may lead to frequent hunger and difficulty managing weight. We will delve further into how different types of hormones impact various body systems including the immune system, endocrine system, and the gut. Finally, understanding these signs and symptoms is vital in identifying potential hormonal imbalances and seeking appropriate treatment.

Most women will not need to worry about the issues we are about to discuss; however, they are still worth understanding. I've personally struggled with premenstrual dysphoric disorder (PMDD), which was plaguing my mental health. I was at work with two female coworkers when one of them told me to "stop being dramatic" when I asked to go home. The physical and mental pain was so bad. Fortunately, my other coworker understood how difficult periods can be. While she did not know anything about premenstrual dysphoric disorder (PMDD), she took the time to listen, even leaving halfway through her shift to get me some painkillers.

Owing to the fact that so much information exists, it is easy to get confused or to misunderstand some very important things.

The Problem of Self-Diagnosis

Something I feel we need to address is the growing trend of self-diagnosis. I'm not saying that self-diagnosis is wrong or inherently invalid because, under the right circumstances, it can be validating and empowering. However, all too often I see women diagnosing themselves with a variety of disorders that they don't fully understand.

When it comes to hormonal imbalance and hormone disorders, misinformation can lead to dire consequences like autoimmune diseases such as Hashimoto's disease. Hashimoto's causes the thyroid to malfunction, which can lead to hyperactivity or underactivity.

Hashimoto's disease is an endocrine disorder with a very specific set of diagnostic criteria, and it's very easy to look at a set of criteria and check "Yes" to all.

However, that's where the problems come in: With self-diagnosis comes self-treatment. While an internet search can help find information and a sense of community, it's also a hotbed of advertising and misinformation. If you search, "Hashimoto's natural treatment," the first result is a sponsored banner of supplements that claim to help with Hashimoto's symptoms. There are also a variety of blog posts, websites, and articles, some of which are well-researched, and others are clearly trying to sell you something.

One of the problems with self-diagnosis is that it's often not accurate. A 2019 study reported that "patients are not accurate reporters of their own history of some autoimmune diseases" (O'Rourke et al., 2019). It's possible to spot the signs and symptoms, which is what this chapter is about, and draw conclusions from them, but if the conclusion you draw is incorrect, it can have negative consequences.

In some cases, people might feel a little bloated after eating a lot of carbohydrates. That's not unusual; carbohydrates can cause you to retain water. However, those people might see bloating as a sign that they have celiac disease or another form of gluten intolerance. They would then cut out all carbohydrates from their diet, maybe going on a high fat, high protein diet without understanding how those diets work, and subsequently end up in the hospital with kidney stones or ketoacidosis (a condition where there are so many ketone bodies in the blood that it becomes acidic).

This is why I am so fervent about speaking to a medical professional and advocating for yourself. If you have to ask to see a female doctor or a doctor who identifies as a woman, do it. Self-diagnosis can be validating and empowering, but only when you have the right information and proper tools with which to do so. The process for a formal diagnosis is long and painstaking, not only because of the paperwork involved but also because of the extensive testing that needs to be done. However, it will all be worth it to finally have answers.

The Wide-Ranging Signs and Symptoms of Hormonal Imbalances

In this section, we are going to look at how hormones affect the body and some of the most common signs of female hormonal imbalances. In line with the previous section, please be aware that the purpose of this section is to give you an idea of what hormonal imbalances could look like, and how they could feel. You might experience some of these symptoms yourself, but that doesn't mean you have the condition mentioned. If, however, you suspect that you might have it, get yourself to an endocrinologist as soon as you can.

How Hormones Affect the Body

A hormonal imbalance occurs when your glands produce too much or not enough of their particular hormones. Depending on the hormone in question, you will experience different symptoms. For example, an excess of androgens in women can cause excess facial hair, which can be treated with medication or through laser hair removal. You might notice changes in your weight (either weight gain or weight loss), a reduced sex drive, and possibly acne, but this depends on the hormone that is out of balance.

Hormonal imbalances can have a variety of effects on the body. Some affect your physical appearance and sex drive, as described above. Other imbalances can affect your background systems, such as digestion, sleep, and your immune system.

Digestive disruptions include:

- Tachycardia (fast heartbeat)
- Unexpected weight gain or weight loss
- Lethargy or fatigue
- Diarrhea, frequent bowel movements, or constipation
- Numbness or a pins and needles sensation in your hands and feet

- Elevated blood cholesterol

- Depression or anxiety

Your circadian rhythm is your sleep cycle. We need the sleep cycle to ensure adequate rest after a busy day. Hormones fluctuate throughout the day, the most important in this case being melatonin. Melatonin is the sleep hormone, and it is released in response to certain stimuli. For example, when it starts getting dark outside during the winter months, we might feel tired a lot earlier than in the summer. In warmer months, we might feel lethargic and in need of a nice nap. When melatonin is in balance, you will get adequate sleep and awaken feeling rested and energized.

There are many reasons why your sleep cycle might be disrupted. Sleep apnea is a condition where, during sleep, breathing sporadically stops and starts. It can be dangerous and can cause you to lose sleep if you suffer from it. Narcolepsy is another sleep disorder characterized by sudden bouts of sleepiness, where you can fall asleep at any time without warning. A more commonly known condition is insomnia, which is the inability to fall asleep or sleep for long enough periods of time to feel rested.

There are other conditions that can cause an imbalance in the circadian rhythm, but these are the most common. If you struggle with your sleep schedule, it would be worth speaking to a medical professional.

Disruptions to your sleep cycle can also be very dangerous. A prospective study found that sleep deprivation "is associated with a substantial increase in risk of motor vehicle crashes in the general population" (Gottlieb et al., 2018). Furthermore, a report by the National Sleep Foundation found that "drowsy driving-related motor vehicle crashes account for roughly 20% of all motor vehicle crashes" (*Frequency of Fatigue-Related Crashes,* n.d.). This is not just limited to car or road incidents. If you are deprived of sleep, you should avoid operating heavy machinery, lifting heavy objects, and cleaning. Instead, seek professional help to regulate your sleeping pattern.

Sleep cycle disruptions include:

- Sluggishness or lethargy
- Difficulty falling asleep
- Increased blood pressure
- Changes in mood
- Weakened immune system

Your immune system is the reason you don't get too sick too often. Infections happen all the time, and your immune system is constantly fighting them off. One of the reasons we have technology, such as the flu vaccine, is to give the immune system a little extra help during flu season. Hormonal balance is crucial to keeping the immune system functioning. A regular sleep pattern, for example, allows the body to rest and heal from the day before, giving the immune system a chance to break down and dispose of anything you picked up throughout the day. Or, if you do get sick, it gives your body some much-needed time to fight the infection.

Three hormones play a vital role in keeping the immune system functioning: estrogen, progesterone, and androgens (okay, that last one is a group of hormones). Even men have small amounts of estrogen and progesterone that function to support a healthy immune system. Estrogen is probably the most important, as estrogen deficiency "is associated with reductions in cell mediators involved in the inflammatory response. Aging itself is associated with chronic inflammation" (*Could Hormone Replacement Therapy Boost Your Immune System?* 2020).

Immune system disruptions include:

- Inflammation (in severe cases, this can be chronic)
- Cell dysfunction
- Cell and tissue damage
- Onset of autoimmune conditions, such as chronic fatigue or arthritis

We talked briefly about estrogen and how it is a key hormone to the immune system, ready to fight off anything that it doesn't recognize as part of the body. In autoimmune disorders, however, the immune system effectively attacks itself.

When there is an estrogen deficiency, such as in perimenopause or menopause, the immune system takes a hit. In the days leading up to your period, you might notice that you experience cold or flu-like symptoms a bit easier. This is because your estrogen levels fall during the menstrual cycle, specifically just after ovulation when your body is preparing for pregnancy and your immune system needs to be able to allow sperm through for fertilization to occur.

How to Identify Hormonal Imbalances

Hormonal imbalance looks different in everyone, although there are a few key signs to keep a lookout for. The signs and symptoms listed below are worth keeping an eye on:

- Heavy or painful periods

- Unexplained weight gain or loss
- Skin problems, such as acne breakouts
- Fertility problems
- Headaches or migraines

If you experience any of these, speak to a medical professional as soon as possible. While some of the signs and symptoms we've covered in this section seem ordinary, they can be the warning signs of something more severe. Ask for a referral to an endocrinologist and tell them everything in detail. For example, if you experience long periods, note whether this runs in your family history or if this isn't normal for you. Advocate for yourself and make yourself heard.

By working with a healthcare professional, such as an endocrinologist, you have access to a variety of tests that can get to the root cause of the problem. The symptoms are only a part of it, and once you know what the cause of it all is, you can take action and bring balance to your hormones.

A Holistic Approach

When you hear the words "a holistic" approach you might think of a group of people living away from society and subsisting on roots and water. This is not the case. A holistic approach to health is simply seeing all parts of your health—mental, emotional, and physical—as a single unit. When one is out of balance, all of them are out of balance. There are a few things you can do to bring your health into alignment using a holistic approach. You don't have to move into the woods and live off the land, but you do have to take a step back and examine the choices you are making.

Start Making Changes

The best way to start on a holistic health journey is to make lifestyle changes. Lifestyle changes include, but are not limited to:

- Increasing daily physical activity

- Avoiding unhealthy foods

- Limiting the amount of refined or processed sugar in your diet

- Drinking more water

- Going for more walks in nature

- Implementing a self-care routine (such as yoga, a regular massage, or aromatherapy)

- Taking up journaling

- Finding a creative hobby, such as reading, dancing, or painting

By finding new hobbies and implementing changes to your lifestyle, you are subtly manipulating your brain chemistry. Creative hobbies, such as dancing, release serotonin and dopamine, the "feel good" and "reward" hormones. During times such as PMS, perimenopause, and menopause, serotonin and dopamine are sorely needed and difficult to come by. While these hobbies might be something of a distraction, it is a necessary distraction and one that can pay off in the long run.

If you want to make changes to your diet, start by limiting the amount of caffeine and sugar you consume. I love a cup of coffee or tea every so often; it helps me feel human, especially on a Monday. However, caffeine works by stimulating the pituitary gland, which responds by signaling an emergency to the adrenal glands, which then produce adrenaline, thus, leaving you depleted and dehydrated. A diet full of excess sugar also increases the chances of insulin resistance and the onset of type 1 diabetes (the diabetes which is influenced by lifestyle factors). By doing this, you can help bring balance to your insulin levels, as well as your pituitary gland and adrenaline.

Managing Your Hormone Health More Effectively

Managing your hormone health is not easy. Habit formation requires behavior change, and that behavior change has to be the result of consistent practice and boundary-setting. When you finally get the hang of it, your hormones and your health will thank you. I'm going to offer a few tips on how to more effectively handle your hormone health.

The first thing to do is to get into a routine, which makes it much easier to maintain homeostasis, and what state does the body love being in? Homeostasis. Your body loves to know when you're going to wake up, when you're going to eat next, when you're going to bed, and when you're going to have that next cup of coffee. You get the picture: The body loves routine, and so does homeostasis.

Second, practice mindfulness. Mindfulness is the purposeful ability to bring your attention to the present, without judgment or preconceived notions. This is a skill that can be developed and cultivated through regular meditation as well as mindfulness training. You can practice this in daily life by reducing your screen time, journaling your experiences, and noticing the space that you are in.

Third, breathe. It sounds obvious; breathing happens automatically after all. In yoga, breathwork is referred to as "pranayama," which can be translated as, "breath control" or "breath restraint." Prana is the vital life energy that flows through every living thing, although you might see it referred to as "breath." That's what we're working with here: breath. Simple breathing techniques have been shown to greatly reduce anxiety by slowing the heart rate, which signals to the pituitary gland that all is safe. Try this simple breathing exercise:

Equal Breath

- Find a comfortable position, seated or lying down, whichever you find most relaxing. If it helps, you can light a candle or some incense. Take notice of how you are feeling. Anxious? Jittery? Uncomfortable?

- Settle into your natural breath. Notice the length and quality of your inhales and exhales. Take in cool air on the way in, and warm air on the way out.

- Slowly empty your lungs. On your next inhale, breathe in for a count of two. Your next exhale should also be for a count of two. Take as many rounds as feels comfortable.

- Gradually increase your inhales and exhales to a count of three, and then four. Again, take as many rounds as you feel comfortable. You do not have to stick with a count of four if it is uncomfortable; a count of two is fine.

- If you want to take it further, you can inhale for a count of three, while exhaling for a count of four.

- Slowly, come back to your natural breath, and notice how you are feeling.

There are many breathing exercises you can do to slow down your heart rate; this is just one of my favorites. While yoga and breathwork cannot cure everything, they can go a long way to alleviate some of the negative side effects of hormone imbalance.

Conclusion

Hormonal imbalances occur for many different reasons and in many different ways, ranging from subtle symptoms to severe health issues. Signs and symptoms can look like anything. They can be as simple as feeling tired a little earlier than usual, or you could be experiencing something ongoing. Hormonal imbalances are not always something to worry about. They can occur throughout the day since it's a normal part of homeostasis. When our blood sugar gets low, glucagon is released to stabilize it, and when we get hungry, the body releases ghrelin to signal that it's time to eat. Without these naturally occurring imbalances, the body cannot function. We will discuss when you should consult a doctor in a later chapter.

Self-diagnosis can be a valuable tool and even a good jumping-off point, but it can also be dangerous. Unless you have all the information you need at your disposal, including (but not limited to) a complete family history of diagnosis, a thorough understanding of the diagnosis you are seeking, and a list of other possible conditions, you could end up doing more harm than good. Many women fall into the trap of misinformation. We are a prime target for various companies selling a myriad of herbal supplements and the like, all in an effort to make a profit. Herbal supplements do have their place, but they are not to be the only cure.

There are many ways to maintain your hormonal health at home. For example, if you know your diet isn't the best, taking a multivitamin can be helpful to "top up" what you are missing.

Vegetarians and vegans, for example, tend to be quite low in iron and B12, so a multivitamin can be helpful. Nutrition also plays a key role in hormone balance, which is something we will look at a little later on.

If you miss a night or two of good quality sleep, chances are you will feel a bit drowsy and struggle throughout the next day, so as long as you catch up on your sleep and remain consistent with your sleep cycle, you will be fine. The sleep cycle is also not the only system that can be affected. When out of balance, your immune system can begin to falter, allowing in pathogens that can cause you to get sick. By recognizing these signs, it will aid in the early detection and management of hormone imbalances. The symptoms will largely be dictated by the respective roles the hormones play in the body. A holistic approach, considering multiple factors, is necessary to balance hormones, as hormonal health affects—and is affected by—overall well-being.

Chapter 4:

Causes of Hormonal Imbalances

A whole host of things can cause hormonal imbalances. Hormones are cyclical, notable examples include the sleep cycle and the menstrual cycle. However, there are other factors that can cause hormonal imbalances. These factors can be broken down into genetic conditions and lifestyle factors.

Genetic Conditions

There is a present genetic component to many hormonal conditions. Some conditions, such as diabetes, have different categories. Type 1 diabetes is influenced by lifestyle factors, gestational diabetes develops during pregnancy (and usually clears up in the time after birth), and type 2 diabetes is genetic. If your family has a history of diabetes, you are more likely to develop it yourself. It is also important to note that, just because something is genetic or has a genetic component, it doesn't automatically mean that you *will* develop it. It just means that your likelihood of developing it has increased. For example, it's entirely possible to have two parents who carry the gene for Hashimoto's so their children's *likelihood* of developing Hashimoto's later in life is increased. Note that "increased chance" does not mean "will definitely develop."

Genetic hormone balance conditions include (but are not limited to):

- Type 2 diabetes

- Polycystic ovary syndrome (PCOS)

- Hashimoto's disease (Note: Although Hashimoto's disease tends to be genetic, some cases are not hereditary)

What Is a Hereditary Disease?

A hereditary disease is a category of diseases that are the result of changes in a person's DNA, also referred to as genetic disorders or inherited diseases. These include:

- Type 2 diabetes

- High blood pressure (genes likely play a role)

- Some forms of cancer

- Hemophilia (a blood clotting disorder)

- Cystic fibrosis

Genetic diseases have been the subject of focus for a very long time. One of the earliest observations was in 1902 when Archibald E. Garrod published a study suggesting that alkaptonuria (also known as black urine disease, where the patient produces black urine) might be the result of a recessive gene (Urban, 1999). In 1988, "it was found that, before approximately age 25 years, greater than or equal to 53/1,000 live-born individuals can be expected to have diseases with an important genetic component" (Baird et al., 1988). And, more recently, a paper was published highlighting the research to date on the genetic model of hereditary diseases (Hieter et al., 2023). Thanks to research, we learn more every year.

Diseases might be considered hereditary if more than one person in your family has the disease. For example, epilepsy might "run in the family" if your mother, one of her siblings, and one of your grandparents has the condition. Some diseases can also "skip a generation." These are referred to as autosomal recessive diseases, and they equally affect men and women. Usually, "generational skipping" occurs when the generation after the affected generation is unaffected. To use the epilepsy example, your mother might have epilepsy, but you do not. Therefore, in this case, you are the generation that epilepsy has "skipped," but you are a carrier for it.

Just because a disease runs in your family doesn't mean it's a death sentence. Some cancers are hereditary, but advances in medical technology have made it possible for patients to not only beat their cancer but recover and live full lives. Other diseases, unfortunately, don't have this same outcome and people's everyday lives have to be shifted to accommodate the disease, like cystic fibrosis, which affects the lungs.

What to Do If a Disease Runs in Your Family

Assuming that a genetic disease runs in your family, what do you do about it?

The short answer is: Get tested, and if you have it, treat it.

The long answer is: Speak with your doctor and determine your risk. Once you are aware of the risk, if you do not have the disease, take reasonable measures to prevent the disease from developing in the first place. Of course, as with anything, the disease might still develop, and you will have only succeeded in delaying its development. If you are lucky and it never develops due to your preventative efforts, you can go about life as normal.

When you see your doctor, they can recommend any number of changes. They might recommend a preventative course of medication, changes to your lifestyle, or even recommend that you do nothing differently and, instead, worry about it when the time comes. This last one is the case for many people. As with some diseases, no matter how hard you try to prevent them, they can and will develop no matter what. All we can do is face them on our feet.

Type 2 Diabetes

A well-known genetic condition is type 2 diabetes, which is a metabolic condition characterized by elevated blood sugar levels. If left untreated, it can cause health problems. Common health problems associated with diabetes include diabetic ketoacidosis and diabetic coma. Diabetic ketoacidosis occurs when there is a high presence of ketone bodies in the blood, causing the blood to turn acidic. A diabetic coma occurs when blood sugar levels are so high that the body has no option but to shut down. Treatments for diabetes include medications, such as insulin and metformin (the main first-line medication), and lifestyle changes, such as a healthier eating pattern and exercise.

At present, it is understood that there is no "diabetes gene." Rather, only certain genes are involved with the onset of diabetes, specifically the TCF7L2 and ABCC8 genes. TCF7L2 affects the production of glucose and the secretion of insulin, while ABCC8 regulates insulin. Genetic mutations can occur at any time, not just before you're born or when you're conceived. Some environmental factors can influence your genetics, even while you're walking down the street! These factors include the climate, pollution levels in your local area and even your access to nutritious food and physical activity.

Your genetics are not set in stone. They govern how you look, and your likelihood of developing diabetes, but there's only so far your genetics can take you. Mutations in specific genes can cause, or increase the likelihood of, the development of diabetes. Each mutation, no matter how small, can have large consequences. The two genes mentioned above, TCF7L2 and ABCC8, are only two of the numerous genes affected.

Diabetes is a metabolic condition, and it affects all of the body's metabolic processes. By extension, diabetes also affects a diabetic woman's hormonal balance, specifically because the ovaries might mature faster, which can lead to early perimenopause and menopause.

Polycystic Ovary Syndrome

Polycystic ovary syndrome (PCOS) causes cysts to grow on the ovaries. While there is a genetic component to this condition, it is estimated that it is largely environmental. A 2019 literature review suggests that higher androgen levels during gestation might influence the onset of PCOS later in life (Khan et al., 2019). However, many studies we have surrounding this theory are based on animal models, specifically sheep, rats, and monkeys. This is due to ethical barriers surrounding human experimentation.

Although it is unclear what genes play a role in the onset of PCOS, it is clear that, like diabetes, certain mutations may hold an influence. These mutations result in certain risk markers, such as promotor pentanucleotide (TTTTA)n polymorphism which is a genetic predisposition factor for PCOS (Bhimwal et al., 2023). In biology, polymorphism occurs when there is more than one copy of something. In the case of PCOS, the clue is in the name: cysts.

Polycystic ovary syndrome (PCOS) can affect the balance of reproductive hormones by producing excess amounts of androgens such as testosterone. This can lead to painful, irregular periods and fertility issues.

Hashimoto's Disease

Hashimoto's disease is another common condition with a genetic component. Much like diabetes, if you have family members who have it, then it is possible that it runs in your family. Genes and traits do not "skip" generations; they lie dormant until they are, if at all, activated through a series of genetic and environmental factors. Hashimoto's is thought to be one such condition. Although no specific genes have been identified as the "Hashimoto's gene," it is a mutation of a gene family that is believed to be the cause. This gene family is the human leukocyte antigen (HLA) complex, which plays a role in regulating the immune system and protecting it from pathogens, such as viruses and bacteria. Hashimoto's disease is a disease that affects the thyroid, and it is possible that mutations in the HLA gene family cause the immune system to attack the thyroid.

Other factors, besides genetics, are believed to influence the development of Hashimoto's, like sex. Most people who develop Hashimoto's are women, although the reasons for this are not clear. It is believed that the mutation occurs on the X chromosome, of which women have two copies. Another theory is that women's immune systems are more reactive than men's. Additionally, Hashimoto's disease tends to develop between the ages of 30 and 50, with symptoms worsening as th thyroid progressively deteriorates.

Another factor is diet. We will cover nutrition in a later chapter, but for now, there are a few minerals that are vital to thyroid function: selenium, zinc, and iodine. While the human body needs these in small amounts, it is possible to be deficient in one or more of them. This is why some treatments include the supplementation of iodine, zinc, and selenium.

Although the symptoms of Hashimoto's disease are not unique and can be mistaken for other conditions, you should still be aware of them. The symptoms include:

- Hair loss

- Slower heart rate

- Increased sensitivity to temperature

- Muscle cramps

- Constipation

- Unexplained weight gain

- Amenorrhea or irregular menstrual cycle

- Fatigue

- Goiter (a growth on the thyroid)

Given that Hashimoto's disease is a condition of the thyroid, a deficiency in thyroid hormones can cause irregular periods. This can also lead to infertility issues.

Lifestyle Factors: Diet, Exercise, Stress, and Sleep

In addition to genetic factors, there are also a variety of lifestyle factors that can increase the likelihood of genetic conditions developing. These factors include your diet, exercise, physical activity, levels of stress, and even your sleep cycle. The body is a biomechanical marvel that will do anything to keep itself alive and awake when you are, so it will do a lot of things in order to maintain homeostasis. This includes moderating hormone secretion and reactivity. If you are drinking coffee, your body will produce more adrenaline in response to your caffeine intake. Similarly, if you are settling in to go to bed, your pituitary gland will secrete melatonin to help you feel sleepy.

These are just a couple of ways your body responds to external stimuli. Let's have a look at how these stimuli influence your hormones in a little more detail.

Diet

Your body has a set of systems in place to maintain homeostasis, and in order to do that, it has a very specific set of hormones that regulate the digestive system and the digestion process. In fact, there are 10 hormones that govern digestion. The body knows what it's doing in order to maintain homeostasis. When we eat food or drink a beverage, it can have a direct effect on how hormones are secreted. This can be through simply entering the gut. Secretin is then released. This hormone has three functions:

- Regulation of gastric acid

- Regulation of pancreatic bicarbonate

- Osmoregulation (maintaining the balance between salt and water in the body)

When we eat, acid secretion is at its highest. When we are not eating, acid levels are at their lowest. After food has been digested, the pancreas releases pancreatic bicarbonate in order to neutralize excess stomach acid (Miraglia et al., 2018). When we use the washroom, there are traces of stomach acid, along with bases such as bicarbonate (pancreatic and sodium) that neutralize the pH, so the average bowel movement of a healthy person is around 6.6—a little acidic. For context, the human body's pH is slightly alkaline at 7.3–7.4.

Another way one's diet affects hormone health is the insulin response. When we eat food, particularly carbohydrates (sugars), the body releases insulin, which breaks down glucose. Try this experiment: Take your blood sugar before a meal and let half an hour go by. Then, take your blood sugar again. Don't be alarmed! The rise you are seeing is perfectly normal. 30–45 minutes after you have finished eating is when blood glucose is at its highest saturation. If you take your blood sugar for a third time, around an hour later, your levels will most likely be back to normal.

Poor diet and an unhealthy lifestyle can affect the way your hormones are produced and utilized throughout the body. By getting regular movement and eating a balanced diet, you will be helping your hormones take care of themselves. In Chapter 7, we will look at this a little more closely.

Exercise

Exercise plays an important role in hormone regulation. No matter what exercise you are doing, you stand to reap all sorts of benefits from it. In terms of hormone regulation, regular physical exercise can decrease the presence of excess sex hormones in women (Ennour-Idrissi et al., 2015). However, there are two hormones that see a slight, temporary increase: testosterone and human growth hormone. They both play a significant role in anabolic processes, such as in muscle growth.

Most women will look at exercise, such as weight training, and recoil because it will "make them look bulky." I assure you that this will not happen. Instead, your muscles will get bigger because you are loading them, and your body will start to look leaner and more toned. In fact, by exercising—no matter what kind—you are improving the balance of your reproductive hormones. One study showed that estrogen levels and symptoms of estrogen-dominant conditions, such as PCOS, improved after exercise (Woodward et al., 2020).

During exercise, you are using glucose which has been stored in your muscles. This stored form of glucose is called glycogen, and it's stored in the muscles as an extra source of fuel for when you're in a fasted state, such as sleeping. Glycogen is released from the muscles and converted into glucose, which is used to give you energy during your workout. Because you are burning glucose while exercising, you are not using insulin. This is why in the time after you've finished a workout, insulin levels tend to be lower.

Overexercising, on the other hand, can lead to a condition called chronic stress. Although stress is not inherently bad, extended periods of stress can have negative side effects. Extended periods of exercise can cause excessive production of endorphins (adrenaline and cortisol, among others), leading to inflammation and dysregulation in your hormonal balance.

Sleep

The circadian rhythm is a series of mental, physical, and behavioral changes that occur in 24-hour cycles. These changes have several key roles in the body, including hormone secretion, hunger and fullness cues, digestion, body temperature, and sleep. Like all other hormonal processes in the body, the circadian rhythm loves routine. It likes knowing when you are going to go to bed and waking up; it likes knowing when you are going to eat so it can start cueing hunger, and it likes knowing when you're next going to exercise so it can prepare to release endorphins. If your circadian rhythm is disrupted, it can have negative effects on your hormone health. You will become more irritable due to the increased presence of stress hormones, and you will rely on high-calorie and high-sugar foods for quick bursts of energy, causing disruptions in your hormonal balance.

In order to facilitate the sleep-wake cycle portion of the circadian rhythm, your brain needs to secrete a hormone called melatonin, which makes you feel drowsy, lethargic, and ready for sleep. It is released in response to sleep anticipation. External stimuli, such as decreasing daylight or the onset of nighttime, that sleepy-time tea you drink, or even the smell of lavender, can all influence the release of melatonin. Many things can disturb the release of melatonin, including sudden shock, stress, and external factors like loud noises.

A study concluded that "sleep disturbances and, particularly, deprivation are associated with an increased risk of obesity, diabetes and insulin insensitivity, and dysregulation of leptin and ghrelin, which negatively impact human health" (Kim et al., 2015). Sleep deprivation can happen for any reason. It can be the result of stress, or underlying conditions.

Working on your circadian rhythm is simple; you only need to get into a routine. Within a few weeks, this will start to set your internal clock, so your circadian rhythm can release melatonin in order to better facilitate sleep. Also, keep your caffeine intake limited. Caffeine can linger in the body for up to four hours after you've had a cup of tea or coffee. Swap to decaf or herbal tea around five to six hours before going to bed. Limit your screen time, too, by turning off your computer, laptop, television—all of it—and start your evening routine unplugged with some relaxing yoga, breathing exercises, or reading.

Environmental Factors

While it doesn't seem like it at first, there are, in fact, all sorts of environmental or external factors that affect our hormones. We have already explored stress and how it can affect hormone regulation; however, that was from an internal perspective. The stress cycle begins with an *external stressor* and that external stressor can be an environmental factor.

Other environmental factors include endocrine-disrupting chemicals. The Endocrine Society defines endocrine-disrupting chemicals as: "substances in the environment (air, soil, or water supply), food sources, personal care products, and manufactured products that interfere with the normal function of your body's endocrine system" (*Endocrine Disrupting Chemicals,* 2022). Endocrine disruptors can be found in just about anything, including BPA plastics, certain cosmetics that contain parabens, and various pesticides. A 2018 review measuring the presence of endocrine disruptors in hair products for black women found that "hair products tested contained 45 endocrine disrupting or asthma-associated chemicals," (Helm, et al., 2018).

Other factors include pollutants in the air, water, and food. A recent study found a connection between pollution and the development of endometriosis (Vallée et al., 2023). The theory is that pollutants in the air, including carbon monoxide, interrupt the regulation of female sex hormones. In addition, pollution increases the production of stress hormones, which causes us to feel stressed. This constant flood of stress hormones increases inflammation, which can damage the liver and pancreas, as well as other internal organs.

The overuse of medication also influences hormonal balances. Some medications, including antidepressants, work by increasing the availability of certain hormones. Selective serotonin reuptake inhibitors (SSRIs) increase the availability of serotonin. However, addiction to—or reliance on—medications can damage hormone receptors. For example, consistently taking stimulants can overwork and damage the adrenal glands, causing mood and anxiety disorders.

Moving from hair care to cleaning, let's discuss how endocrine disruptors end up in our daily lives. If you have ever worked in a kitchen or other food service environment, you have probably worked with heavy-duty cleaning chemicals that require all sorts of personal protective equipment (PPE). This is because those cleaning chemicals are carcinogenic, meaning they can cause cancer. Synthetic cleaning products, especially heavy-duty ones, can mimic our naturally occurring hormones, which can disrupt the body's sense of homeostasis.

Conclusion

Hormonal imbalances can stem from a multitude of sources, including physiological conditions, environmental factors, and lifestyle choices. Understanding these causes necessitates a broad approach to maintaining hormonal balance. Simply addressing one factor without considering others might not effectively restore hormonal health. Every woman's hormonal balance is unique, influenced by her own unique combination of these factors.

Recognizing the diverse causes of hormonal imbalance provides valuable insights into the interconnected nature of the mind and body, paving the way for the following chapter on comprehensive lifestyle, diet interventions, and medical interventions to restore hormonal balance. The wide range of causal factors we have discussed in this chapter highlights the importance of personalized hormonal care and leads to the next chapter on tailored hormonal management strategies. We also need to be aware of environmental factors and hidden dangers in everyday products to further investigate our daily routines and choices.

There are numerous factors that can cause hormonal imbalances in women, ranging from physiological, environmental, and lifestyle-related contributors. These factors can distress the endocrine system and disrupt hormonal balance. Physiologically, conditions such as polycystic ovary syndrome (PCOS), thyroid disorders, diabetes, adrenal fatigue, and pituitary tumors can impede the proper functioning of the hormonal system. Environmental factors also play a role in disrupting hormonal balance, including chemicals found in many common household products. Finally, lifestyle-related causes, such as the impact of stress, lack of sleep, poor diet, insufficient physical activity, and obesity all have an effect on hormonal health.

Chapter 5:

Effects of Hormonal Imbalances

Most of the symptoms we have covered so far can be due to hormonal imbalances, but they can also be completely normal consequences of bodily functions. Eating too much can result in bloating while doing too much exercise can result in chronic aches and pains. This is why pursuing the input of medical professionals is so important—it removes all other possibilities and gets to the heart of the problem. Hormonal imbalances can have severe effects on daily life, most of which cannot be resolved by simply drinking a glass of water.

Hormonal imbalances have a variety of effects. Some of them affect us physically, while others affect us mentally or spiritually. In this section, we are going to explore a few of these effects, as well as some ways you can deal with them when they arise.

Impact on Physical Health

One of the most common physical effects of hormone imbalance is weight gain. Weight gain happens when we eat too much and move too little. This is referred to as a calorie surplus. When our hormones are out of balance, like when we're stressed, we find ourselves craving high-calorie foods. We also might find ourselves with an insatiable hunger, finding it difficult to shed fat and gain muscle. The resulting stress causes us to overeat and gain weight.

Weight fluctuations appear to happen overnight. If you have trouble sleeping, weigh yourself the next morning; you might find that you have gained weight. Meanwhile, if you weigh yourself in the morning after a full night's sleep, you might find that you've lost weight. A regular sleep schedule has been shown to help regulate your appetite (Dashti et al., 2015). Sleeping is essential time for the body to recover and restore itself after a long day. If we don't get that energy from sleep, we need to find it elsewhere, and that elsewhere is a higher caloric intake. An adequate length of sleep affects the ghrelin and leptin hormones. The less sleep we get, the more ghrelin the body produces in order to make up for the loss of energy. The more and better quality of sleep we get, the more leptin is produced, which means that we have fewer hunger cues and are less likely to eat an excess number of calories.

Another way hormone imbalances can affect our physical health is through the onset of chronic disease. Chronic fatigue syndrome has no single cause. Bacterial infections, nerve damage, mental illness, and hormonal imbalance have all been linked to the onset of chronic fatigue syndrome. The hormonal link is through the thyroid gland, and if the thyroid is overactive or underactive, it can cause fatigue. This is most often seen in women. As the thyroid regulates the body's metabolism, if it is over or under-working, this can result in a disruption in how the body uses energy.

Impacts on Mental and Emotional Health

One of the worst things about premenstrual syndrome (PMS) and premenstrual dysphoric disorder (PMDD) is how much they screw with your mental and emotional health. If you have PMS, you might feel a little down and disoriented, and you might cramp up a little more than usual. If you suffer from PMDD, there is a good chance that you will question your self-worth, be unable to move, and be unable to focus on being productive. Some women find that their thoughts turn to violence during bouts of PMDD.

Speaking from personal experience, I have found that taking supplements like zinc, iron, B12, and magnesium has done wonders for me and how I react during different times in my menstrual cycle. During menstruation, the body will use a lot more of these minerals than it will on a normal day, which means that it will be out of balance. This includes the hormones it uses to metabolize these minerals.

One of the worst struggles women face when dealing with hormonal imbalances is that they are not taken seriously. They might be brushed off for being "a drama queen" or dismissed as being "just on their period." This is nonsense, of course, because only *you* understand when something is wrong. This is when it begins to affect your well-being and way of life.

Well-Being and Quality of Life

Having hormonal imbalances can drastically affect your way of life. Endometriosis causes tissue similar to that of the uterine lining to grow outside of the uterus. This can cause extreme pain and heavy periods, and in some cases can even be fatal. On the less extreme (yet still drastic) end, some women get periods that are so bad that they are unable to leave the house. Menopause can have a similar effect. The hormonal fluctuations during these two critical hormonal stages in a woman's life can be so volatile that it is difficult to plan or predict one day from the next.

Other conditions, such as polycystic ovary syndrome (PCOS), can cause physical issues which may leave a woman feeling embarrassed or unwilling to leave the house. One of these is facial hair growth. While PCOS is rapidly becoming more visible and better understood, there still exist people who treat women with PCOS as targets. This is, of course, unacceptable, and this sort of behavior is why many women with PCOS find it difficult to step out of the house. There is hope, however, as PCOS does have a broad range of treatments that can make it more bearable to be outside and interact with others.

Early Detection and Mitigation

Detecting symptoms early can be a huge advantage in the fight for hormonal balance and overall well-being.

Waiting for symptoms to appear is a sign that you have waited too long, and now all you can do is manage the condition. Alzheimer's takes root between the ages of 30 and 40, and the symptoms start to show in your 50s and 60s. It is not impossible to detect Alzheimer's early in life or to take preventative measures. However, because the symptoms appear so late, all you can really do is take steps to manage them, hoping to buy yourself some time. This is why early detection and mitigation are so important. It doesn't just apply to a condition like Alzheimer's. Any condition, be it diabetes, PCOS, or endometriosis, can benefit from early detection.

Mitigation is simply taking preventative measures. If you go to the doctor, they might be able to give you a list of recommendations for mitigating any hormonal conditions that may arise in the future, including anything from preventative medicine to increasing your physical activity or making changes to your diet. Some doctors may be unwilling to refer you for anything on the basis of age or sex, but this is why we need to advocate for ourselves.

Early detection also has its issues. A 2016 study found that "if documentation protocols are not established and followed, early detection systems could expose both individual clinicians as well as healthcare institutions to medical–legal risk" (Escobar et al., 2016). Let's put this into context. Let's assume that a thyroid condition runs in your family, so you are at risk of developing it too. You go to your doctor and they confirm that, yes, you could develop it, but it's nothing to worry about "right now," and you're safe to go about living your life until you need to take action. Fast forward a few years and you have developed the condition. Your new doctor tells you that when you went to the doctor and were informed that you could develop it, that was the "ideal time" to start taking preventative action. This puts the first doctor at fault, and they can be sued for medical negligence.

Another issue with early detection is that you might become paranoid or worry too much about potentially developing a condition. I see this a lot in my friends. Some of them are at risk of developing type 2 diabetes because it runs in their families, so they start doing everything they can to prevent it from happening. This results in some extreme measures. Some people take to the keto or carnivore diet because they are both low-carb diets that don't cause insulin spikes. Others wear constant glucose monitors (CGMs) even though they don't have diabetes yet. I often look at the women in my life and wonder, "Are you being smart about early detection and mitigation, or are you taking it a step too far?" There's no way to know for certain, but I do encourage you to be educated before you take any preventative measures.

Conclusion

Hormonal imbalances affect us in more ways than we think. When a woman is having her period, she is brushed off as "emotional," and while she is emotional, it's not without reason. Her pain is as real as the pain of a broken leg.

Chapter 6:

Hormones and Nutrition

Hormones and nutrition go well together. In addition to our sex and growth hormones, we have hormones that are primed to help the body absorb different nutrients. We have already talked extensively about ghrelin and leptin—the hunger and fullness hormones—but there are so many others. Different nutrients can influence hormone production and regulation. Certain types of foods may stimulate or suppress the release of particular hormones, ultimately impacting health. For instance, carbohydrates affect insulin levels, and fatty acids influence sex hormones. A balanced diet is key to maintaining hormonal equilibrium. However, there are some problems we cannot avoid when it comes to hormone balance. Overnutrition and malnutrition, for example, are easy ways to throw your hormones off. There's also the problem of extreme dieting, all of which we will look at in due course. First, let's take a look at some of the nutritional hormones.

The Nutritional Hormones

Ghrelin

This is the hunger hormone. When the stomach is empty, it releases ghrelin, which makes its way into the bloodstream and up to the brain. Ghrelin then acts on the hypothalamus to signal that we are hungry. This results in us feeling that the stomach is empty, along with the stomach rumbling. The more ghrelin there is in the bloodstream and acting on the hypothalamus, the hungrier we get. Ghrelin assists with the regulation of energy balance in the body, only ceasing to be produced when we are getting full. It also stimulates the production of growth hormones by acting on the pituitary gland.

Leptin

This is the "fullness" hormone. Although leptin is released to signal when we're full, its main function is to alter food intake and regulate energy expenditure. You can find leptin stored in adipose tissue (body fat) and fat cells. When leptin is released, it enters the bloodstream and, like ghrelin, it acts on the hypothalamus, which is a small area in the center of the brain that helps to produce hormones that regulate the heart rate, body temperature, hunger levels, and the sleep-wake cycle.

Gastrointestinal Hormones

Gastrointestinal hormones are umbrella terms used to describe a group of chemical messengers that facilitate many functions in the gastrointestinal tract. They govern many digestive processes including the secretion of ghrelin and stomach acid, aiding the digestion of solid food, furthering the absorption of nutrients, and enabling gut motility such as gastric emptying.

Insulin

Diabetics may be familiar with insulin. Insulin is the hormone that regulates the body's blood sugar. It allows blood sugar to be absorbed into the body so that it can be used as a source of energy. Additionally, insulin signals to the liver to store sugar for later use.

Glucagon

Glucagon is secreted by the pancreas to regulate blood sugar levels. When it is present in the blood, your blood sugar levels increase.

The Problem of Extreme Dieting

There is nothing wrong with going on a diet. In fact, in many cases, changing your diet can have a lot of health benefits. Extreme dieting, on the other hand, can have negative consequences on our bodies and our hormonal balance. Take the example of cholesterol. There are two types: low-density lipoprotein (LDL) cholesterol and high-density lipoprotein (HDL) cholesterol, where HDL cholesterol is the "good" cholesterol. However, cholesterol in general has a lot of negativity surrounding it because high levels of LDL ("bad") cholesterol can lead to cardiovascular health problems, like heart attacks, strokes, and angina. Due to this negative press, there has been a significant rise in diet trends determined to cut cholesterol-containing foods out of the picture.

When I say "extreme diet," I am talking about diets that remove entire food groups. The ketogenic diet severely restricts carbohydrates, while the carnivore diet cuts out all plant-based foods and focuses entirely on animal products, such as meat, dairy, fish, and eggs. These diets are unsustainable and are often portrayed as being "the key to weight loss." The result is that the dieter will lose weight, only to gain it back once coming off of the diet.

Take the keto diet: Due to the extreme limitations on carbohydrates, insulin production and regulation are severely affected. Ketogenesis is the body's way of producing energy from dietary fat in times when carbohydrates are not available. It's supposed to be a temporary solution to a temporary problem. However, when you come off the diet after sustaining it for a long period of time, the body will immediately revert back to using carbohydrates for fuel. It will also hold onto whatever it can of its favorite energy source. As a result, you will go back on keto, and enter into a cycle of yo-yo dieting.

And that's just the keto diet. There are plenty more that I can go into, and they all have the same effect: They impact the endocrine system. The body responds physically and physiologically to extreme and crash diets. You may have heard of starvation mode. Starvation mode is the name given to the mode your body employs when it's not getting enough energy. This reduces the number of calories it needs to keep functioning, lowering the basal metabolic rate.

The best thing you can do for your hormones, through your diet, is to focus on a diet rich in whole foods, with a minimal intake of processed foods. Focus on the quality of food you're putting into your body. The better you nourish your body, the better your hormones will balance.

Nutrients and How They Affect Your Hormones

Nutrition is vital to health, and without proper nutrition, we risk our health falling into imbalance. Across the world, there is massive nutritional disparity. In the United States, we have more than enough to go around, not just of healthy foods, but of all types of processed junk too. Processed junk food can be okay in moderation, but the average American diet is made up of 73% ultra-processed junk (Nowell, 2023).

"Ultra-processed" here refers to food items that are made from substances extracted from foods, such as starches, fats, and added sugars. All food goes through a process. An apple farmer picking an apple off a tree has put the apple through a process, getting it from the tree to your kitchen. This is not the same process that ground meat goes through in order to become a hamburger. The excess of ultra-processed junk has taken a significant toll on the nation's health, and it is beginning to burst at the seams.

Micronutrients

Micronutrients play vital roles in the body's maintenance and metabolism, "including enabling the body to produce enzymes, hormones and other substances needed for normal growth and development" (*Micronutrients*, n.d.). Micronutrients are just vitamins and minerals which can be found in the food we eat. Vitamin C supports the immune system, calcium supports healthy bones, iron supports red blood cell development, and B12 (niacin) supports DNA replication. There are 27 different types of micronutrients, and as the name implies, they are small compared to macronutrients.

Macronutrients generally contain some or all of the micronutrients. For example, oranges and lemons are often listed as great sources of vitamin C, and that's completely true. Oranges and lemons are high in carbohydrates, the body's favorite macronutrient and its preferred source of fuel. When these carbohydrates are broken down in the digestive system, they are broken down into all of the micronutrients they contain, and the body begins to utilize them right away.

Micronutrients work on a small scale to help us regulate our hormones. The body produces some hormones specifically to metabolize various nutrients. This can be thrown out of balance by two simple things: overnutrition and malnutrition.

Overnutrition

Overnutrition is an imbalanced nutrition intake characterized by an excessive intake of nutrients that impairs health. This can be a symptom of orthorexia, an eating disorder whereby the patient is obsessed with eating only the healthiest foods to the point that they have a list of "safe" foods they eat from. Additionally, a person may become overnourished if they partake in excessive multivitamin consumption. Multivitamins can be helpful, but studies show that you're really just paying for expensive pee (Jia et al., 2022).

There *are* cases where multivitamins can be helpful. If you have received bariatric surgery, such as a gastric bypass, multivitamins can increase the nutritional quality of your diet. On the other hand, if you do not need multivitamins, you could be doing more harm to your body than you think. A 2018 study found that in patients who suffered from obesity, overnutrition actually *inhibited* leptin production and its actions on the hypothalamus (Fruwürth et al., 2018). Leptin, as you may recall, is the hormone that is released to signal fullness. If leptin is not released, hunger cues will continue, leading to overeating.

Overeating can lead to obesity, which can cause hormonal imbalances. These include estrogen deficiency, iron deficiency anemia, and growth hormone deficiency.

Malnutrition

Malnutrition is an imbalance characterized by not getting enough of the nutrients you need to remain healthy. This can be a symptom of anorexia, an eating disorder where the patient intentionally undereats with the goal of losing weight. Like orthorexia, the patient may have a list of "safe" foods or unusual justifications for not eating certain foods. Malnourishment also occurs in several parts of the world where there is a drought, social unrest, or simply not enough food to go around.

Like overnourishment, malnourishment can damage our bodies but in more obvious ways. The first sign is typically excessive weight loss, although there are cases where being malnourished can cause weight gain. Eating a diet high in ultra-processed foods that contain very little in the way of nutrients can lead to the body being nutritionally hungry, while you are still consuming excess calories. Another symptom is vitamin and mineral deficiency. Iron deficiency anemia is among the most common deficiencies, along with vitamin C, B12 (niacin), and magnesium deficiencies.

Iron deficiency anemia and B12 deficiency anemia are characterized by low iron or low levels of B12 presence in blood, and symptoms include fatigue, weakness, pica (a condition where you might crave non-food items such as coal or bricks), and cloudy thinking. Vitamin C deficiency can lead to scurvy, although the first symptoms of this are usually lethargy, weakness, irritability, and weight loss. The hormones responsible for metabolizing iron are called hepcidin, so in problems like iron deficiency anemia, the production of hepcidin is limited.

So, how does malnutrition affect our hormones? Because we are not getting enough of what we need, the body starts to slow itself down. This is due to the thyroid producing less hormones in order to reduce the body's basal metabolic rate (BMR).

Conclusion

Nutrition and hormones go hand in hand. The body has numerous processes to keep everything in homeostasis, that perfect state of balance. Without the proper nutrients received from a balanced diet, the body cannot produce the hormones required in sufficient quantities. Proper nutrition is, therefore, key to this. Eating plenty of lean meats and a variety of grains and vegetables will provide your body with what it needs. Be mindful of supplements. While they can be helpful and a "top up" of sorts, taking too many can cause issues, such as iron toxicity. If this happens, speak to a doctor right away.

Chapter 7:

Lifestyle Management for Hormone Health

A balanced lifestyle is essential for optimal hormonal health. Beyond nutritional factors, the role of regular exercise, stress management, sleep patterns, and environmental factors all add up in their influence on the endocrine system. For instance, chronic stress can upset cortisol levels, and regular exercise helps maintain insulin sensitivity. Lifestyle disorders, like obesity and diabetes, are also detrimental to hormonal balance. In this chapter, we are going to explore some strategies to manage your lifestyle, with the aim of achieving a balanced hormonal state.

Stress

Just to clarify something: You can influence certain hormones through your diet, but you cannot change your body's pH. The pH of the body ranges from 7.35 to 7.45, so the body likes to be a little more alkaline. If your pH drops below 7.35, you are at risk of acidosis, a condition where your body becomes acidic and effectively starts digesting itself (*Acidosis,* 2021).

The reason I bring this up is simple: When folks start learning about hormone balance, they learn how interconnected everything is. They also start to think that the food we eat and the beverages we drink affect the overall pH of the body. This is not the case. You can influence the pH of the stomach by eating because the stomach needs to be acidic in order to facilitate digestion. Your blood can become acidic through a condition like ketoacidosis. You cannot enter a "fat-burning" or "hormone-balancing" zone just by changing your diet.

As we saw, your diet can affect the balance of your hormones. Insulin, ghrelin, and the rest of the digestive hormones are the hormones that are affected. There are several hormones that regulate your body's pH. One of the key hormones that does this is aldosterone which is secreted from the adrenal glands— the same glands that produce cortisol and adrenaline. Its main role is to regulate the levels of electrolytes in the blood, which includes sodium.

Something we don't often acknowledge, let alone talk about, is the stress response. The stress response is the sum of the body's internal and external responses to stressful stimuli. These responses can include an elevated heart rate, dilated pupils, sweating, shallow breathing, muscle aches, headaches, and difficulty sleeping. The stress response is a part of the stress cycle, of which there are five stages: external stimulus (also called the external stressor), internal appraisal, physiological response, internalization, and coping.

1. *External Stimulus/Stressor*: This entails the stimulus that causes you to feel stressed. For example, when you get to work, you see that you have received an email letting you know that you have to meet with HR later that afternoon.

2. *Internal Appraisal*: You start trying to reason what the meeting could be about. You try to tell yourself that it might be something positive, such as a pay raise, but you think of all the worst-case scenarios, such as a potential layoff.

3. *Physiological Response*: Your body starts to respond to the stress, and you experience the symptoms we covered earlier.

4. *Internalization*: Humans think in a story, and it's at this point in the stress cycle that we have constructed that story. Perhaps it's along the lines of, "I accidentally drank my boss's coffee on Friday and now I'm getting fired."

5. *Coping*: You brace yourself for the worst-case scenario and try to calm yourself down as best you can.

Stress affects the way hormones are secreted, and the level of each hormone in the blood. The culprits, and I use that word lightly, are cortisol and adrenaline, which are necessary—I cannot stress that enough. The role of cortisol is to regulate the stress response, and the role of adrenaline is to help keep your heart beating and your lungs breathing. It is perfectly healthy to have cortisol and adrenaline in the blood. However, it is not healthy to have consistently elevated levels of cortisol and adrenaline in your blood.

Extended periods of elevated cortisol and adrenaline are referred to as chronic stress. Symptoms of chronic stress include aches and pains, sleepiness, insomnia, cloudy thinking, increased recreational drug and alcohol use, overeating, low energy, emotional dysregulation, change in behavior and attitude toward others, and change in social behavior (for example, a normally extroverted person might become more introverted). Long-term effects can cause hypertension (high blood pressure), cardiac arrest, strokes, and inflammation of the circulatory system. Chronic stress can also lead to sleep deprivation, which we will cover in the next section.

Dealing with stress sounds easier than it is. One of the first things I recommend is finding a quiet space to sit and practice breathing exercises, such as the "Equal Breath" exercise we practiced in Chapter 3. This will help bring down your heart rate and may relieve some of the tension in your muscles. Another thing I recommend, especially for work-related stress, is making use of your paid time off and sick days. According to a study by Statista, in 2022, 26% of Americans between 18 and 65 years old did not take a sick day (Elflein, 2023). There is a slight aversion to using your sick days, but I promise you this: You come first.

Different Types of Stress

Stress is a perfectly normal bodily phenomenon. The body needs stress in order to remain balanced. When we exercise, the body experiences physical stress and responds by making us stronger, healthier, and able to endure more. Stress can be emotional or physical. If you are waiting on an important email from work, that's emotional stress; if you are ill while doing squats at the gym, that's physical stress.

Stress is a reaction. Specifically, it occurs when the body is meeting a challenge or a demand that it is unfamiliar with. Stress is not always a bad thing and can be good in certain circumstances. When humans were evolving, stress helped us avoid danger by giving us the ability to run away quickly. Nowadays, we might use stress to help us get to work on time or to meet a deadline at work or school. Problems arise when stress overstays its welcome, becoming chronic.

There are four types of stress: acute, chronic, episodic, and eustress.

Acute stress is short-term, leaving as quickly as it comes. We typically experience this type of stress when we're in the midst of an argument with our loved ones or when we have to come to a sudden stop in traffic. If you're a thrill seeker, you might experience this kind of stress while bungee jumping. Everyone experiences acute stress.

Chronic stress is long-term. It can last for days, weeks, or even months at a time, and usually occurs as a result of long-term issues; for example, you might experience chronic stress if you have had student loans for a long period of time or are stuck in a relationship or friendship that no longer serves you. If the thing causing you stress goes on for an extended period, your stress will go on for an extended period. The unnerving thing about chronic stress is that you become used to it. So used to it, in fact, that you forget you are stressed to begin with.

Episodic stress, sometimes referred to as *episodic acute stress*, occurs when you frequently experience periods of acute stress. You might always feel like something is about to go wrong or that you're always "on the go" and under pressure to get things done.

Eustress is a beneficial type of stress. It's an underlying, consistent stress that the body needs in order to perform necessary functions, such as keeping the immune system active, facilitating the heartbeat, and regulating energy efficiency. It's a sort of baseline type of stress if you will.

Stress is not inherently a bad thing; it's just a response to a stimulus. It only becomes a problem when it begins to affect our daily lives. It can also cause a phenomenon referred to as "adrenal fatigue." Although this is not a medical diagnosis, it is the name given to feeling tired from being so stressed. This is because cortisol, the stress hormone, is being produced in such vast quantities from the adrenal glands that we no longer feel it. This is when we need to implement techniques and strategies to manage our stress so that it stops affecting us so harshly and doesn't affect those around us.

Stress Management: Tips, Tricks, and Techniques

Breathing exercises are an effective way to reduce stress, especially exercises that focus on extending the exhale. Controlled breathing, in this manner, signals to the body that you are not in danger. Stress can be a response to danger, which can result in acute, chronic, and episodic stress. By slowing down your exhales, you will lower your heart rate and, therefore, your blood pressure. This tells the body that it's okay to relax. You are moving your body from "fight or flight" to "rest and digest."

It also helps to take control of what is making you stressed. You cannot control the events that make you stressed, but you can control your response to them. If you are having financial problems and are putting off looking at or paying your bills, then allot some time to sitting down and going through your finances. See where you can cut back, and how you can collate any debts you have. If you are struggling with work, delegate some of your responsibilities or prioritize them. You do not need to take on the weight of the world.

Guided meditation also helps to alleviate stress. When you get stressed, your mind becomes a jumble of thoughts related to everything you have to do, and everything that makes you stressed. By listening to a guided meditation, you are focusing your attention on the person speaking and the imagery of the meditation, which helps to relax the mind and relieve stress.

If you can afford it or can find a good deal, treat yourself to a deep tissue massage. The body holds onto tension, which causes physical stress. Think of how your jaw clenches or how your shoulders go up to your ears. A deep tissue massage works into the fascia—the three-dimensional webbing that glues the muscle to the bone—and untangles knots in the muscles. This releases tension, allowing you to be more relaxed.

Another way to manage stress is by physically exercising. We will be looking at exercise in more depth later, but for now, let's focus on how it can help you with stress.

Some sports, such as boxing and powerlifting, allow you to relieve any aggression associated with stress. Both of these sports, and exercise in general, allow the parasympathetic nervous system (rest and digest) to release the hormones dopamine and serotonin. While this happens, the body also decreases the production and presence of cortisol and adrenaline.

You can also try yoga. There are many different kinds of yoga, although the three that are ideal for stress are Ashtanga, Vinyasa, and restorative. Ashtanga is all about moving seamlessly between the poses, and there is no energy to waste or time to think, so it's great for getting your mind off of what's stressing you out and focusing on the flow. Vinyasa flow yoga is all about linking breath to movement, with a heavy emphasis on breathing techniques to slow down your rate of exhale. Yin yoga is more meditative where you hold the poses for longer than you would in Vinyasa, which allows the body to unknot itself and relax.

Cultivating a Healthy Environment

When we talk about hormonal balance and health, we talk about the key things: getting enough sleep, exercise, and nutrients. Those things are all important, there's no denying that. However, we rarely talk about the environment we find ourselves in. That could be our work environments, our homes, the streets we live on, and even our social media spaces. Humans are social creatures, and we constantly pick up subtle cues from all around, which influence the way we think and behave.

A healthy environment looks different for everyone. For some, it's getting enough sleep, waking up at 7 a.m., and eating a balanced diet. For others, it's waking up at 4 a.m., getting enough protein, and meditating for three hours. We all have our own version of balance, and how to achieve it. A healthy environment is characterized by how much it nourishes us, and how much it encourages us to engage in healthy behaviors. If you live with someone who regularly puts you down, this will discourage you from pursuing healthy habits. On the other hand, if you live with someone who is always encouraging you, this will motivate you to adopt and maintain healthy habits.

Maintaining a Healthy Sleep Schedule

When we covered the circadian rhythm in a previous chapter, it was in preparation for this section. Maintaining a healthy sleep schedule is as vital to your hormonal health as anything else you do. If you sleep well, your body is better equipped to produce and use the hormones it needs. If you get poor sleep, your body limits the production of some hormones in favor of others, as it prioritizes maintaining adequate levels of energy.

According to the National Institutes of Health, 40% of American adults fall asleep during the day, and up to 19% of those did not get adequate sleep (*What Are Sleep Deprivation and Deficiency?* 2022). Reasons for this include being surrounded by distractions, being unable to settle the mind, having too much caffeine throughout the day, and simply not feeling tired.

In order to talk about maintaining a healthy sleep schedule, it is important that you first start by creating a healthy sleep schedule. Maintaining something requires it to be a habit first, so get into the habit of going to bed at a reasonable time. This will be easier when it's wintertime, depending on where you are in the world. In winter, the days are shorter and nights are longer, so take advantage of that and train yourself to go to bed at a reasonable time (say, 9 or 10 in the evening). Within a few weeks, you will naturally start feeling tired at your new bedtime.

Another thing to try is ridding yourself of all distractions. Your phone will have a "sleep mode" setting, or it will allow you to schedule some screen time limits. Set your screen time to end about half an hour before you go to bed. This will allow your mind to properly decompress and start to settle down. The sleep mode setting will turn the light on your phone from white spectrum light, which is visually stimulating, to blue spectrum, which is visibly calming.

One more thing you can do is limit your caffeine intake in the hours before going to bed. Caffeine lingers in the system for between four to six hours, depending on how much you have ingested. The recommended daily allowance is no more than 400 mg of caffeine per day, although many Americans exceed this dose due to long work hours (*Spilling the Beans: How Much Caffeine Is Too Much?* n.d.). If you drink a high or moderate dose of caffeine a few hours before bed, you might find that you have a difficult time getting to sleep. This is because caffeine blocks inhibition, which means that melatonin (sleep hormone) production is limited. Instead of caffeinated beverages, opt for the decaf version, herbal teas, or plain water.

A Balanced Diet

We covered the importance of nutrition and how it relates to hormones in a previous chapter, so now let's briefly discuss the benefits of a balanced diet. When we talk about a "balanced diet," we are talking about an equal distribution of micronutrients and macronutrients as a way of maintaining our health. Each body has its own unique needs. No two people will, for example, respond to carbohydrates in the same way. Some might get an intense sugar spike within 30 minutes of eating a croissant, while others will hardly feel anything.

A balanced diet can yield many benefits, from improved digestion to potentially helping you live longer. You might hear the term "eat the rainbow" when researching helpful tips on how to eat a balanced diet, which refers to eating a variety of fruits and vegetables, all of which have different nutrient profiles. A nutrient profile is simply an explanation of what nutrients are in that particular food, and it's also why "superfoods" are not a real thing. Blueberries and strawberries are just as rich in nutrients as acai berries, and bananas are as equally good a source of potassium as avocados.

Another thing to watch out for is marketing gimmicks. I used the term "superfood" because this is a popular buzzword to describe a variety of otherwise ordinary foods that have a higher-than-average concentration of certain nutrients. Acai berries, for example, contain a slightly higher concentration of antioxidants than other berries. Avocados are rich in unsaturated or heart-healthy fats. However, it is possible to have too much of a good thing. For example, vitamin C is great for maintaining the immune system and helping the body absorb nutrients like calcium and magnesium, but getting too much of it can cause nausea and diarrhea. Iron helps red blood cells produce hemoglobin, which carries oxygen throughout the body. If you get too much iron, you can develop iron toxicity, also called iron poisoning, which can cause black and bloody stools, nausea, abdominal pain, and it can even lead to liver damage in extreme cases.

A balanced diet is vital to attain balanced hormones. Getting just the right amount of macro and micronutrients will not only fuel the body but will also help to regulate the hormones required to metabolize them.

Maintaining Movement

Just like not getting enough nutrients can lead to an imbalance in your hormones, being overweight or underweight can cause the same thing. Being overweight can cause a high body temperature, which can make for an undesirable environment for your hormones. Your hormones will denature, which will make them ineffective or function inadequately. Conversely, being underweight will cause a body temperature that is too low. As the body puts more energy into staying warm and keeping the vital organs (heart, lungs, and brain) alive, it expends less energy on less important tasks, such as reproductive hormones.

A sedentary lifestyle can occur for any reason. You might be experiencing a case of depression so severe that it prevents you from getting up and moving or causes mobility issues, resulting in your lack of desire to move. There are numerous dangers to living a sedentary lifestyle, including weight gain, increased risk of cancer, osteoporosis, increased risk of metabolic diseases such as dyslipidemia and diabetes mellitus, cardiovascular disease, and many more. A sedentary lifestyle is not healthy and cannot be made healthy. This is why it's important to find a way to be—and stay—active.

You don't need to go to the gym in order to increase your activity, although that is an option. There's something called NEAT: Non-exercise activity thermogenesis. This is energy produced or calories burned at active periods during the day. NEAT activities include things like going for a walk, doing chores, or simply getting up and stretching. It's nothing fancy, and it's nothing too complicated. It is simply finding ways in your daily life to increase your movement. Below are some ways to increase your NEAT:

- Take up a new hobby, something that gets you up and moving

- Walk to the grocery store and carry your groceries home

- Fidget more often—keep your hands and feet moving

- Avoid taking the bus for short distances—choose to walk instead

- Take the stairs where reasonable (Note: You do not have to climb 50 flights of stairs, just whatever you can manage)

Now that we have covered ways to increase your NEAT, or non-gym activities, let's talk about going to the gym and being active.

There's such a thing as "gymtimidation," which is simply being intimidated by going to the gym. If you want to go to the gym, there's a simple solution to getting over your nerves: Ask for help. You might be surprised to learn that personal trainers are there to help, and they're usually around and available to help during gym opening hours, specifically to help members. Gyms usually offer classes that aim to teach you how to exercise, taking you through basic movements with the goal of improving your understanding of your body and the exercise itself.

Depending on the gym, you will also find several pieces of equipment that might look more like medieval torture equipment to you. If you ask a personal trainer to take you around and show you how to use the equipment that scares (or confuses) you the most, you will have a much easier time at the gym.

Regular Exercise: Strength and Cardio

There are many different kinds of exercise—you most likely see new trends every day. At the time of writing this book, the exercise trend everyone is talking about is bouldering—or indoor rock climbing. It's a great exercise for people who want to develop their arm strength and core stability, but depending on where you go, it can be expensive. That's why it's important to find local group fitness classes to attend, particularly cardio and strength training.

"Cardio" is short for "cardiovascular," as it refers to the heart and lungs. It is helpful to develop your ability to breathe and reduce breathlessness. Regular cardio has been shown to improve the body's ability to use oxygen, which results in reduced strain on the heart, so it doesn't need to pump as hard to get blood around the body. Common cardio exercises include running, walking, swimming, cycling, stationary cycling, indoor rowing machines, dancing, and boxing.

Strength training, also referred to as strength and conditioning, is a type of training focused on developing muscles. There are different kinds of strength exercises, some of which can be performed with only your body weight, such as squats, lunges, and high planks. These exercises can also be performed with added weight in the form of dumbbells, barbells, medicine balls or, if it's all you have, a sack of flour. Strength training has been shown to increase muscle volume and tone, which improves overall mobility. Women shy away from strength training because it can be seen as "manly," but it's really not. It's just a way of maintaining your muscles. As we age, and as our hormone levels change, muscle tone begins to atrophy—wither away—which increases the risk of falls and injury in old age.

If you do not want to get into strength sports or go hard in the gym, find local classes. Functional strength classes are what I recommend for beginners, and they focus exactly on that:

functional strength. These classes are ideal for people who want to become more confident and comfortable in the way they move and feel within their bodies. You might feel nervous in your first class, but I encourage you to keep going. You will soon find that others are there for the same reason you are: to get stronger. Expect a lot of lunges to work the glutes and quadriceps, isometric holds to strengthen the core, and push-ups to develop the back.

Stretching and Strengthening: Yoga and Pilates

Yoga is a strengthening practice. Depending on the type of yoga, you can expect different benefits. The more active styles such as Ashtanga and Vinyasa are great for developing a connection with the breath and body, while Bikram yoga is great for working up a sweat. Yoga is also great for developing balance. In addition to the major muscles—the glutes, pectorals, quadriceps, etc.—the body has a network of stabilizer muscles. Yoga balances, such as tree pose or one-legged chair pose, are especially good for training the stabilizers.

Yoga allows your parasympathetic nervous system to activate. You are so focused on not falling in a balance, or keeping pace with the rest of the class, that your body spends its nervous energy on maintaining your focus.

It is impossible to find a yogi who looks like a bodybuilder unless you know a bodybuilder who does yoga, but that's not to say that yoga doesn't make you strong. Yoga poses require you to engage your muscles. Think of it as a series of body weight movements that are sequenced together with a focus. Some flows are focused on opening the chest and improving mobility in the shoulders, while others have a theme such as grounding or balancing.

Pilates is more of a challenge. Yoga is full-body focused, even when there's an anatomical theme. When you take a Pilates class, you are focusing on building strength, toning your muscles, and strengthening your core.

Conclusion

Making changes to your lifestyle is never easy. Once something is a habit, it can be difficult to break. Breaking a habit requires a good deal of willpower that not many people are able to cultivate. However, if you are able to discipline yourself enough to make the changes required for the sake of your hormonal health, the benefits can be great. Increasing your physical activity is one of the best things you can do for your hormonal health because it helps to regulate various systems in your body; in particular, the central nervous system, the immune system, and the insulin response. Mindful practices, such as yoga and Pilates, are also good for toning the body and improving overall well-being.

You should also be aware of the role your environment plays in your hormonal health. I don't just mean what it's like at home, I mean your general surroundings. Pollution and climate change play a big role in health in general. If you live in a crowded city, you are exposed to thousands of airborne toxins every day, along with the stress of having to survive in that city. If it benefits you, and you are able to, find somewhere green with lots of fresh air, as this will help to reduce your stress levels, and by extension, restore balance to your hormones.

Chapter 8:

Natural Remedies and Supplements for Hormonal Health

Natural remedies have been around for a very long time, so long in fact that herbal treatments were an early form of medication. Many of these are still in use today; for example, medieval Arab doctors would prescribe a plant-based diet to their patients to improve their digestion and health. The popular appeal of herbal remedies and natural remedies is that they are natural.

As civilization developed and grew, so did our understanding of the human body and how it works. We came to understand that "natural" does not always mean "safe." After all, cyanide is naturally occurring and can be found in apple seeds and bamboo shoots. Don't fret about that, though—you would have to eat so many apple seeds or bamboo shoots that it wouldn't be worth the effort. Arsenic is also naturally occurring and can be found in shrimp. Again, you would have to eat tons of them in order to ingest a lethal dose.

Some natural remedies are also not great for certain conditions. St. John's wort can be used to alleviate the symptoms of anxiety and depression. This is because it acts in a similar way to a selective serotonin reuptake inhibitor (SSRI, a widely used antidepressant) and increases the availability of serotonin and other neurotransmitters. However, St John's wort is also not recommended for asthmatics or people with other lung conditions because it can cause symptoms to worsen and, in some cases, cause asthma attacks.

In this chapter, we will delve into the realm of natural remedies and supplements for hormonal health, with a focus on current scientific findings. Various herbs, plants, foods, and supplements will be explored in relation to their influence on hormonal health. We will also briefly examine the role of adaptogens like ashwagandha and rhodiola in stress and hormonal balance. Adaptogens are natural supplements that help the body adapt to stress.

Supplements: The Science

To put it simply, *most* people are wasting their money on supplements. In many cases, they are buying supplements they don't need. In other cases, they are buying multiple supplements, only some of which they need, when they could be purchasing a single multivitamin. The supplement market is huge and difficult to navigate. The trick lies in knowing what you need and why you need it. If you need an iron supplement because it helps to alleviate menstrual pain every month, then take an iron supplement. If you need to take a calcium supplement because you can't eat dairy, take a calcium supplement.

The most basic natural remedy or supplement is your diet. Nutrient deficiencies can occur for any reason. Perhaps your body doesn't absorb magnesium properly, or perhaps you're among the almost 50% of Americans who don't get their recommended intake of magnesium (Razzaque, 2018). By incorporating more nutrient-dense foods into your diet, you will generally be getting everything you need. Nutrient-dense foods include kale, spinach, avocado, whole grains, eggs, lean meats, nuts, and legumes.

One of the hang-ups about herbal supplements is that the side effects are both common and rare, and patients might also not report them to their doctor when seeking medical support. As many herbal supplements can interact with other medications, it is important to state that they are being used (Furhad & Bokhari, 2023). Additionally, a 2021 comprehensive study found that there is limited efficacy in taking over-the-counter herbal supplements (Bessell et al., 2021).

So, what does this mean? It just means you need to be sure you're taking your supplements for the right reason, and in your case, it's for hormonal balance. During some of the more hormonally unbalanced times of a woman's life, such as during pre-menstrual stress or menopause, supplements can be helpful. Iron supplements or evening primrose oil can be helpful for premenstrual stress, while black cohosh can be helpful for menopause. While the evidence is still being gathered, the interest in black cohosh is due to an extract found in Remifemin, which can decrease symptoms of menopause.

Adaptogens

An adaptogen is an herbal substance that can help the body adapt to stress. This can be any type of stress like oxidative stress or stress from waiting on a text from your partner. Think of them as herbal anxiety remedies. Some are more effective than others, although there are three that, in general, are considered to be quite useful: ashwagandha, aloe vera, and rhodiola. While there are several studies that discuss the limits of herbal adaptogens, there are several studies into the three named adaptogens that offer promising results. In this context, we are talking about feeling stressed, not oxidative stress.

Adaptogens such as ashwagandha and rhodiola have shown promise in helping the body adapt to stress and in maintaining hormonal balance. By incorporating these remedies into your daily routine, you can expect them to contribute to hormonal harmony. Bear in mind that what works for one person might not be suitable for you. This is why a personalized and holistic supplementation strategy is vital for optimal benefits, considering individual dietary patterns and lifestyle factors. It is important to always place an emphasis on maintaining a healthy and balanced diet, getting enough exercise, and finding peace in your mental health.

The use of these herbal remedies has been shown to reduce the effect of stress in humans, as we will now explore.

Ashwagandha

Ashwagandha comes from a shrub native to India. When taken as a supplement, the extract is taken from the root. It can be taken in pill form, other times as a liquid to swallow. Ashwagandha came onto the scene as a buzzword, sort of like a superfood that can "calm the brain, reduce swelling, lower blood pressure, and alter the immune system" (Leal, 2020). As quickly as it appeared on the scene, it disappeared and is now uttered in wellness circles by people who are trying to sell you an overpriced supplement. Despite this, ashwagandha has been shown to have some positive effects on hormone health, particularly in relation to stress. A study found that the use of ashwagandha "as a supplement for stress and anxiety management could be an excellent alternative option" (Salve et al., 2019).

Aloe Vera

Aloe vera is a type of succulent plant—you might have one in your bathroom for an added splash of greenery. Don't eat it though, edible aloe vera is different from the plant you have in your bathroom. If you browse the shelves at your local health food store, you might find edible aloe vera products, like gels, juices, capsules, and maybe some skincare products, such as face masks and creams. Aloe vera has many uses because it's an adaptogen and is full of healthy sugars and antioxidants.

Aloe vera can be just as effective in reducing menstrual pain as ibuprofen (Sardashti et al., 2020). One of the theories surrounding this is that aloe vera is under the category of "phytoestrogen." Phytoestrogen is a compound that mimics the behaviors of estrogen found in the body. Depending on the purity of the gel or aloe vera product you are using, there will be a certain concentration of phytoestrogen in the product, which can have a variety of health benefits, specifically for hormone balance. In addition to reduced menstrual pain, symptoms of menopause can also be reduced, along with decreased risk of cardiovascular disease and metabolic syndrome. There are also some non-hormonal benefits; for example, the added fibrous bulk of aloe vera gel can improve bowel movements and be used as a treatment for mild burns.

Rhodiola

One of the latest trends in natural remedies for hormonal imbalance is rhodiola, also known as golden root or king's crown. It can be found growing in high altitudes and has a long history of being used in medical practices across Scandinavia, Russia, and all across Europe. One of its historic uses was as a means to increase performance as well as endurance. Nowadays, it is being used as an herbal remedy for anxiety and depression, and to improve athletic performance. At present, there is very little in-depth research into rhodiola, although what we do have suggests that it can be helpful in treating hormonal imbalances.

It is most effective in reducing stress because just like aloe vera, rhodiola is an adaptogen. A common side effect of stress is a condition called burnout. This occurs when you become so stressed that your body is "running on empty." Rhodiola has a history of being used as a means to improve work performance as well as athletic endurance. Of the few studies we have, one small-scale study examined 118 people who were experiencing burnout from chronic stress, and by the end of the study, all of the participants reported that their burnout symptoms had decreased (Cropley et al., 2015).

Suggested Supplements List

Supplements are precisely what they sound like: They are taken to be an extra source of whichever micro or macronutrient you are lacking. You might need a supplement if you have had bariatric surgery and are unable to eat much. You might need a supplement if you are vegan and not getting enough iron. You might need a supplement if you have been unwell and are losing fluids and, by extension, nutrients. Most people invest in supplements because they believe that they are not getting everything they need in their diet. However, before you start taking supplements, I recommend going to your doctor and getting a blood panel to see if you actually are missing important nutrients in your diet. This will give you an indication of what your diet might be lacking, and you might be able to save a few bucks on over-the-counter supplements by making some changes to your diet.

That being said, some vitamins and minerals can benefit by being supplemented. Below is a list of popular supplements that you might want to consider adding to your diet, assuming that they are needed:

- Vitamin D: Used with calcium for healthy bones

- Omega-3 fatty acids (such as cod liver oil or an omega-3 complex): Joint health and cell formation

- Magnesium: Thyroid health

- Iron: Helps the blood cells create hemoglobin

- B-12 or a B-vitamin complex (a complex includes all of the B vitamins): Great for energy metabolism

- Calcium: Ideal for strong and healthy bones

- Ashwagandha: Overall well-being

- Creatine: Improves energy signaling in the body

- Aloe vera: Menstrual pain relief

- Rhodiola: Stress relief

The Dangers of Supplements

This section is not here to scare you, but it is here to inform you of a condition that can develop. We discussed overnutrition in a previous chapter, and what I am about to discuss with you now is similar to that. Hypervitaminosis is a condition where the body has *too many* vitamins. This condition occurs when the body's stores of vitamins are unusually high. It can be of one particular vitamin, such as vitamin A, or it can be all of them. Whatever the circumstances, it can have potentially disastrous effects.

When the body gets adequate nutrition, it knows what to do. Take calcium, for example. The body metabolizes calcium and stores it in the bones for later use. These calcium stores are constantly in need of replenishment, so if you get enough dairy, or take a multivitamin with some extra calcium, you will be fine. However, if the body suddenly gets five times the recommended intake of calcium per day, it will quickly become unsure what to do with it.

This same thing happens with vitamins. If you get too much of any vitamin, your body will be unable to process it. It will store everything that it is able to and will excrete what it can through urine and feces, but there may still be some left over. Hypervitaminosis can have a wide range of adverse effects on the body. Symptoms include:

- Brittle bones
- Blurry vision
- Migraines
- Decreased appetite
- Changes in alertness

Hypervitaminosis typically happens when you accidentally take too much of a vitamin. Some people are so "on it" with their health that they might take twice the recommended dosage for the multivitamin they are taking. While a multivitamin can be helpful, it can also be harmful. If you are taking any supplements, multivitamins, or anything of the sort, make sure you read the packaging and understand that they are not to be used to replace a healthy, balanced diet.

Conclusion

Natural remedies are not to be used to replace medical treatments. If you want to use them, use them in conjunction with your medication. However, be aware that some natural remedies can have adverse effects on certain medications. While the two most popular natural remedies—aloe vera and rhodiola—are generally quite harmless, I recommend that you spend a good deal of time researching them. Aloe vera is considered to be quite neutral and can even be helpful if you struggle with period pain or are looking for something to supplement your menopause treatment, but not all aloe vera is edible. If you try to eat the gel in the leaves of the plant you have on display in your home, it might not go as well as if you ate some aloe vera gel from your local health food store. Additionally, some natural remedies do not have enough in-depth research. While we do have anecdotal and reviewed evidence that rhodiola can be helpful for stress management, be aware that there is still a lot we do not know.

Chapter 9:

Medical Interventions

Many women dread going to the doctor, particularly for their hormonal health. There are cases where a woman has gone to the doctor for abdominal pain, only to be sent away with painkillers and a pat on the shoulder. Later, that abdominal pain turns out to be endometriosis. Cases like this are why women are now advocating for themselves, taking bolder steps to ensure that they are heard. Menopause can cause depression and anxiety, which can be extreme in many cases, and until recently, there has been little research into how menopause can be treated.

However, when you advocate for yourself, you are capable of getting to the root cause of your pain or your hormonal imbalance. The fact is that you can try all the herbal remedies in the world. You can have the healthiest, most balanced lifestyle possible, and you can still experience hormonal imbalance. This is not the only point at which you should speak with a professional. The earlier you speak with a professional, the sooner you can start building your case and creating a narrative that shows your difficulties have been consistent. But we'll discuss that later.

In this chapter, we are going to discuss modern medical interventions available for women's hormonal health. We will discuss hormonal contraception methods and their impact, hormone replacement therapies, and lifestyle medications, analyzing their pros, cons, and suitability. This chapter also explores surgical interventions, including their risks and benefits. We will also focus on the importance of patient awareness and participation in decision-making processes involving health, and urge for proactive conversations with healthcare providers.

What Medical Interventions Are Available?

The first thing to note is that medical interventions for hormonal health cover a wide spectrum, including hormonal contraceptives, hormone replacement therapies, lifestyle medications, and surgical interventions. Each medical intervention has its own set of advantages, disadvantages, risks, and benefits that require thorough understanding.

One of the first medical interventions a woman might come across is puberty blockers. These have been in the news recently, but rest assured that they are safe, and they have been used for years. There's a condition called precocious puberty, which is when girls as young as eight years old enter puberty early. Precocious puberty is treated with hormone blockers in the early stages because precocious puberty can have adverse effects on a child's body.

Another intervention to consider is hormonal contraceptives. These might be administered when a girl enters sexual development, or they might be administered later in life when a woman begins having sex. Hormonal birth control can come in the form of a daily pill, a monthly injection, or in the form of a topical patch or implant. There are many advantages and disadvantages to hormonal contraceptives. The pros include a reduced risk of pregnancy, it doesn't interrupt sex, periods can be lighter and might be less painful, and some research suggests that it may prevent certain kinds of cancer. The cons to keep in mind are that hormonal contraceptives do not safeguard against sexually transmitted infections, there is an increased chance of yeast infections, a reduced sexual desire, and, in some cases, the formation of blood clots.

In keeping with the theme of contraception, there are some surgical interventions that influence a woman's hormone balance. For example, an oophorectomy is the surgical removal of either one or both ovaries and is typically only done when medically necessary. These cases include women who are at a higher risk of ovarian cancer, women who have diseases such as endometriosis, or when an ovarian cyst is too large to be removed on its own. It is important to note that oophorectomies are not performed as a means of birth control.

Surgical contraceptives, such as a salpingectomy or tubal ligation (getting your "tubes tied"), are also available options. However, these methods are considered permanent or long-lasting. These methods have many advantages; for example, they are very effective in reducing the risk of pregnancy but do not disrupt hormonal balance, so your menstrual cycle continues. However, like with the contraceptive pill, they do not guard against sexually transmitted infections. There are also documented cases of these procedures healing, resulting in pregnancy later in life.

Another hormonal intervention is called the Mirena coil. This is an intrauterine contraceptive device that produces the hormone progestin. The Mirena works by thickening the mucus at the cervix in order to prevent sperm from entering and fertilizing the egg. While the Mirena coil is successful at preventing pregnancy, again, it does not safeguard against sexually transmitted infections, and it can fail close to the end of its lifespan (around five years). When using this, as with using the contraceptive pill or other forms of birth control, consider using a condom if you are having penetrative sex. One disadvantage to consider with the Mirena, as well as other intrauterine devices, is that periods can get worse. Some women feel nothing, others find that their periods stay roughly the same, and a minority find that their periods get significantly worse. Speak with your healthcare provider about whether or not the Mirena is right for you.

Another intervention available to you is hormone replacement therapy, given to cisgender women of menopausal age. It can take the form of estrogen pills, a patch, or a regular injection, and the aim is to alleviate the symptoms of menopause. Estrogen, as well, plays a role in bone density and formation, which is why it's such a vital hormone in women. Some women also take hormone replacement therapy during menopause because it helps them feel "normal" during and after the process.

This is why patient awareness and active participation in healthcare decision-making are fundamental to ensure personalized and appropriate treatment choices. Some people might take to the internet and look for diagnoses that confirm their suspicions. This phenomenon is called confirmation bias. It happens when you seek out information that confirms beliefs you already hold. Confirmation bias, especially when it comes to your personal health and well-being, is not helpful. By looking at different opinions, you gain a broad perspective and a better idea of what to ask about when you speak to your doctor.

So, how can you be as informed as possible when it comes to your hormonal health? It can take up to 90 days to turn a habit into a permanent lifestyle change (Active Iron, 2023). Sexual health clinics exist precisely to inform you of your options when it comes to sexual health. They are also safe spaces where you can discuss your concerns and not be judged. If you think you have a sexually transmitted infection, you will be listened to and assisted. If you think you have endometriosis, you will be listened to and assisted. If you think you have ovarian cancer, you will be listened to and assisted. If you think you are in the early stages of menopause, guess what? You will be listened to and assisted.

How to Advocate for Yourself

You probably came to this chapter expecting me to tell you not to trust your doctor, especially the male doctors who don't know anything about female hormonal health. But you'll find quite the opposite, actually: I encourage you to go to your doctor armed with information and having been to the sexual health clinic already. You want to see an endocrinologist, who spends their life and career studying hormones and hormone health. It's such a nuanced field that we are learning more about it every year, and most of the information is outdated, which is why internet searches can be dangerous.

Internet searches are also why women might be turned away. Women might also be turned away because they're approaching their "time of the month" and whatever pain they're feeling is "normal." A pregnant woman might be turned away for the pain she's feeling in her abdomen as being Braxton-Hicks when, however, it could be more serious, such as a detached placenta. This is why you need to be prepared when going to the doctor.

In this section, I am going to give you the tools you need to better advocate for yourself when you go to the doctor. You might not be going to your doctor for a potentially life-threatening health condition; you might simply be going because you want to change your birth control method but need a doctor's note or a referral for a gynecologist because you want to start having fertility treatments. Whatever your reason for going to the doctor, there are three things you need to keep in mind: your research, what you want to say, and how to challenge a diagnosis that says you're fine.

Be Smart about Your Research

I know what I said about internet searches and cognitive bias, and those things still stand. Much like knowing why you're taking a supplement, you need to be smart about how you do your research. Instead of looking up, "Do I have endometriosis?" search for "endometriosis symptoms," followed by your age range. Also, ask the women in your family—your mother, sisters, aunts, cousins, or anyone who is a blood relative—if they share any symptoms. This will form your family history. Finally, once again, make an appointment at a sexual health clinic with a list of questions. Whoever is there will be able to answer them to the best of their ability.

Write Down What You Want to Say

A lot of women enter the doctor's office knowing what they want to say, but they fumble through it and end up backing out. Write down what you want to say, either on a notepad or in the Notes app on your phone and keep it on hand. Make sure that this list of things to say includes the research that you have done, and what you have done to come by that information. Your doctor may or may not be impressed, but they will be more willing to help you. A doctor's job is very difficult, and you are probably the nth patient your doctor has seen that day, so try and have some patience.

Challenge, Challenge, Challenge

One of the reasons women decide to never go to the doctor is because they are afraid of hearing the word "no." In some cases, this can be life-threatening. If your doctor tells you "No," ask them to make a note in your file saying that they denied taking your case forward to an endocrinologist (or whichever medical specialist you have decided to see). So don't leave until you have seen that your doctor has made that note. This way, you have evidence that you asked, and sometimes, your doctor will relent and refer you to an endocrinologist.

Conclusion

Hopefully, by now, you have a comprehensive understanding of the gamut of medical interventions available for women's hormonal health. Some hormonal interventions, such as puberty blockers in young girls with precocious puberty, have no adverse effects on the patient. As you get older, some hormonal interventions, such as the contraceptive pill, can have adverse effects including making periods worse (such as in the case of the Mirena coil). This, along with the pros and cons of hormonal contraceptives, hormone replacement therapies, and lifestyle medications, will help you better advocate for yourself when you speak with a medical professional.

There are many complexities and potential impacts of surgical interventions on hormonal health to consider, which is why they are often a last resort. Surgery requires preparation and can be expensive as well as dangerous. The role of personal decision-making and open dialogue with healthcare providers is, thus, vital for optimal care.

Chapter 10:

Communicating Hormonal Health Concerns

In the previous chapter, we covered how to advocate for yourself when you go to the doctor. In this chapter, we are going to go a little bit further and cover how to communicate effectively with healthcare providers, while also demystifying certain hormonal health tests. We are going to explore what hormonal health tests are available to you, and how to specify that you want them.

We are going to delve deep into the importance and intricacies of effectively discussing hormonal health concerns. It underscores the significance of transparent communication between patients and healthcare providers, explaining how coherent conversations can lead to precise diagnosis and treatment. My aim here is to provide practical guidance on questions to ask and what symptoms to report, to empower you to openly express your concerns. Furthermore, it's all about communication. There's a lot of stigma surrounding women's hormonal health, and it's about time we start to cut back on some of it.

The Conversation

Let's start with the reason you're reading this chapter: the conversation. In the previous chapter, I gave you some tips: Be smart when you do your research, write down what you want to say, and challenge your doctor if they try to send you on your way.

Clear and candid conversation about hormonal health concerns with healthcare providers is evidently crucial. If you walk into your appointment stumbling over your words or are not clear about why you are there, you will have a higher chance of being dismissed and sent home.

Documenting Your Symptoms

Now it's time to explore how to meticulously document symptoms and appropriately convey them to ensure accurate diagnosis and personalized treatment.

A symptom is a sign of an underlying or apparent disease, but it can also be applied to disorders. Symptoms can be more physical or can be related to mental health issues. Examples include:

- Rashes
- Lumps or bumps
- Unexplained weight changes
- Difficulty sleeping
- Hot flashes

- Fever or chills

When documenting symptoms, be as clear as possible. Write down as much detail as you can, then create a concise description. The description should include the nature of your symptoms, any discolorations that you have noticed, and where your symptom currently is (for example, which body part? Is it on the side of the body?).

Also, keep a note of the time of day. You don't necessarily need the exact hour and minute, but it is important to know roughly when it starts. For example, do your symptoms start in the morning? Or are they more prevalent at night? Do they happen around lunchtime after you've climbed the stairs on the way back to work? When you get out of bed in the morning, do your symptoms feel at their most or least prominent? As your day goes on, make sure to note whether or not they are getting worse or better.

When you speak to your doctor, have your symptom journal on hand. They might flip through it, but they will still make a note of the fact that you have been meticulous in recording your symptoms. This will give your doctor a much better idea of what you are dealing with and how long you have been dealing with it, while also guiding them to the best person to discuss it with. You might be given a physical examination just so they know that the symptoms are there (this has nothing to say about you—it's just so that they can say they've done it and so that they believe you).

Your health is important, but don't rush your symptom journal. Take some time to build it, the same way a lawyer builds a case: With great care, precision, and attention to detail. Around two weeks should be enough to build a good case and fill out your journal, but if you feel you need to take longer, then take all the time you need. If your symptoms have been bugging you for a while but you have never taken the time to journal, make an appointment for a few weeks in the future, and start filling out your journal in the meantime. If your symptoms are new, but still concerning, make the appointment and fill out the journal. Still keep the appointment, even if the symptoms resolve on their own because there's always a chance that they could come back.

The importance of open communication transcends the doctor-patient relationship. It's also a tool to challenge societal stigma around women's hormonal health. You also need to understand the position your doctor is coming from. Your doctor got into medicine to help people—to help *you*—and in order to do that, they spend almost their entire life studying and training just to get their license to be able to sit in that room with you. So, when people say, "What do doctors *really* know?" the answer is, "A great deal, actually." The problem comes from within the infrastructure of the healthcare system. There's a lot of bureaucracy involved including numerous strict policies they have to follow in order to diagnose you or even refer you for tests. Trust me when I say that your doctor is just as frustrated as you are that you're not getting the help you need.

What to Do

In this section, we're going to look at what to do in certain instances. If you are experiencing a hormonal imbalance, these tips and tricks will be helpful in guiding you through how to address them with your doctor.

Menopause and Perimenopause

If you believe you are going through menopause, speak to your doctor and ask for resources on it. An internet search can only help so much in terms of telling you what is happening. When you ask for menopause resources, ask if there is a menopause clinic in your area. A menopause clinic functions similarly to a sexual health clinic but for menopause instead of sexual health. At this clinic, you will have access to hormonal tests that will be able to help diagnose you as being menopausal or perimenopausal. These clinics will also be able to offer all kinds of resources to help see you through the struggle, including hormone replacement therapy.

Hormone Replacement Therapy

Hormone replacement therapy is a form of therapy that aims to replace hormones that are lost or missing in the body. When women go to seek hormone replacement therapy, they might be dismissed on the grounds that their levels are "normal," when, in fact, they might not be. This is usually the case in women with testosterone deficiency, and often with conditions such as PCOS. Many doctors, unless they are specifically trained to become an endocrinologist, will not have had much training in hormones unless they are the basic male and female sex hormones. When asking for hormone replacement therapy, know why you are asking for it. If you suspect that you are menopausal or may have a testosterone deficiency, keep a list of your symptoms and bring it with you to your appointment.

Your doctor might consider prescribing hormone replacement therapy if you are experiencing the following symptoms:

- Night sweats

- Hot flashes

- Change in mood (anxiety, depression)

- Vaginal dryness

- Pain during sexual intercourse

- Lack of a sex drive

- Irregular or no periods (these can occur in women who are not menopausal or perimenopausal)

- Difficulty concentrating

- Weak bones or low bone density

Polycystic Ovary Syndrome (PCOS)

Polycystic ovary syndrome is a hormonal condition that affects the functionality of the ovaries. Symptoms include irregular periods, excess growth of body hair (usually facial), and fertility issues. Treatment is varied and includes medications that limit hair growth and some hormonal replacements to regulate the menstrual cycle. Working to maintain a healthy weight as well as regularly exercising also helps.

When speaking to your doctor about PCOS, you should aim to have the following questions and requests ready to hand:

- Is my thyroid functioning as normal?

- What is my risk of developing diabetes?

- Would it be possible to test my fertility?

- I would like to speak with a specialist.

- I would like you to refer me for an ultrasound. I struggle with losing weight—a calorie deficit and regular exercise have helped me maintain my health but not my weight. Is it likely that I could have PCOS?

One of the symptoms of PCOS is difficulty losing weight, which is why it's more often diagnosed in obese or overweight women than it is in women who are average or underweight. Until recently, it was believed that only overweight or obese women were at risk of developing PCOS, as around 80% of patients who suffered from it were overweight or obese (Sam, 2007). However, we now know that being overweight is not the cause of PCOS, it's more likely to be a symptom.

Take Your Time

Just like we discussed in the previous chapter, write down what you want to say, make a list of your concerns, and bring it to your appointment. Spend a solid amount of time making that list, and don't just search for "hormone imbalance symptoms" online and write those down. Really listen to your body and write down what it's telling you. Write down the symptoms you are experiencing and any hormonal issues (PCOS, Hashimoto's, etc.) that are present in your family. Your appointment is your time just as much as it's your doctor's time. If your appointment time goes over, don't worry, and if this is a concern for you, ask for a longer appointment. Your health is a priority, and you should not be made to feel intimidated or dismissed. Stay calm and persistent if you want to get your questions answered.

Seek a Second Opinion

Do not be afraid to seek a second opinion. It is quite likely that the first doctor you see will dismiss you or view your concerns as hysteria or unfounded. This is where you should ask your doctor to record that they dismissed you. On the other hand, your first doctor might suggest a variety of conditions that could be causing your issues. While this is more helpful than being dismissed, it's always wise to get a second opinion. This way, you have your bases covered in the event that the first opinion is wrong. This is especially true if you feel that you haven't received the care or help you need at the time of going.

Conclusion

Open discussions are of profound significance when discussing hormonal health issues. Every year, doctors face new pressures and must follow increasingly stringent guidelines that block their way to providing adequate healthcare to their patients. The result is usually a short, choppy conversation that leads nowhere. This is why it's important to know who you are talking to, what you are talking about, and why you are talking to them about it. Women's hormonal health issues are often dismissed as "normal" or as "paranoia," but it is possible to push past that and gain some ground when fighting for what you need.

The solution is to cultivate a set of practical skills to convey symptoms and ask pertinent questions to your healthcare providers. Make a list of your symptoms and keep a journal of when you're experiencing them. Understand what the underlying conditions are, but do not go as far as diagnosing yourself with anything. Simply acknowledge that you know you're limited in scope, but you want to take it further to see what can be done.

Finally, a poignant exploration of how communication can aid in defeating the societal stigma rooted in discussions about women's hormonal health is also crucial. There are many barriers to women's health, including stigma. For decades, we've been told that we're "just hormonal" and have had our health concerns pushed to the side because it's easier than dealing with the root cause. By going to your doctor and being open, honest, and candid with them, you can assist in breaking down those barriers and paving the way for more comprehensive women's healthcare.

Chapter 11:

Preventative Measures and Long-Term Maintenance

There's no better cure than prevention. Unfortunately, you can't always prevent the worst, but you can take steps to make it easier in the event of a hormonal imbalance. It's natural to say that hormonal imbalances are going to happen, so prevention and ongoing care play important roles in women's hormonal health. There are plenty of things you can do to maintain hormonal balance, from nutritional adjustments and physical exercises to stress management techniques. Also, do not forget the importance of regular health check-ups and hormonal tests as preventive measures against possible hormonal imbalances.

In this chapter, we are going to look at some things you can do, right now and in the future, to help maintain your hormonal health. All of these things rely on habit formation.

Lifestyle Tweaks

Let's take a look at some tweaks you can make right now to your lifestyle to aid hormonal balance. Some of them are easy to implement while others are a little more challenging. This is why it's important to foster healthy habits.

Building Habits

It can take anywhere from 18 to 254 days to build a new habit (Clear, 2018). You might have also heard of the 21/90 rule: It takes 21 days to make a new habit and 90 days to make it a permanent lifestyle change. Building new habits and lifestyles takes time, so make sure you stay patient. Start small. If you try and do too much at once, you are going to burn yourself out and get very tired of the habit you are trying to build. You do not need to try to build your habit in a day. Your habit will be built over a series of days, with plenty of setbacks and support from others.

While on the topic of setbacks, embrace them when they happen. Habit formation is just as much about learning when you're going too far as it is about building a new lifestyle. When a setback happens, treat it as what it is: a learning opportunity. Something I see a lot when people try to build habits is that they'll naturally stumble and then throw up their hands and say, "I give up." Then, they go right back to being how they were, all of their unhealthy habits intact. Just like a smoker who started smoking at a young age, some habits become intrinsic to us, almost a part of our identity. This is why it's so critical to break this association. Instead of saying, "I'm a failure, and I will always have this habit," it should be, "I had a setback, but cultivating this new habit is important to me."

Habit formation is an uphill battle. It can be difficult, but when you finally crest the top of the hill, the rewards are worth it.

Supplements

While most supplements might not be necessary, there are people who benefit from taking them. Speaking from personal experience, my PMS gets very bad. My cramps are so awful that, sometimes, all I can do is turn off my alarm and stay in bed. I have found that taking iron, B12, zinc, and magnesium supplements has all helped mitigate my pain greatly.

Iron plays an important role in pregnancy and menstruation, which is why you might develop iron deficiency anemia around the time of your period or during pregnancy. As a result, experts suggest that women's iron levels "must be tightly regulated" (Mintz et al., 2020). As we discussed previously, iron is metabolized by the hormone hepcidin. If there's no hepcidin, your blood cells cannot take up oxygen. During menstruation, this is especially bad as the uterus effectively starves itself of oxygen. Iron supplements help by replenishing your stores of iron and preventing heavy menstrual bleeding by aiding in blood clotting.

Magnesium supplements, on the other hand, have been shown to relax smooth muscle (Zhang et al., 2017). As the uterus is made up of smooth muscle that becomes inflamed and starts to cramp during the menstrual cycle, it stands to reason that a little extra magnesium can be helpful.

Physical Activity

To reiterate, "physical activity" does not mean "go to the gym and start busting out reps on all of the machines." Increasing your physical activity just means getting up and moving. This could mean going for a walk, cleaning your house, doing some simple stretching if you are working at a desk, or simply getting up and taking a few steps. Physical activity improves the quality of your muscles and makes it easier to move. This is especially true of activities such as yoga, strength training, and cardio.

Physical activity does not just affect the sex hormones, but it can also help bring balance to your insulin and cortisol levels. During exercise, insulin sensitivity increases, which means that your muscles are better able to receive and utilize glucose during and after exercise. If you work out in a fasted state, or before eating, this will have no effect on how much fat you burn. All it means is that your body is better primed to replenish its glucose stores and to use glucose throughout the day. In addition to regulating insulin, your body also benefits from better regulation of cortisol and adrenaline. Adrenaline and cortisol levels decrease during physical activity, which is why the advice is to "go for a walk" or "try yoga."

Change Your Environment

I'm not telling you to pack up your things and move. When I say "change your environment," it can be as subtle as hanging up some artwork, opening a window, or getting out of the house or away from your office desk. However, if moving is something that you think will help your hormonal balance, then do it. If you live in a city, the stress of the daily hustle and bustle is probably wreaking havoc on your hormones. If you live in the countryside, or somewhere with access to wide, green spaces, you have access to fresh, clean air and nature's greatest resource: the color green.

Colors have different meanings, and green is generally regarded as quite a positive color depending on the shade. Darker greens, such as forest green or grass green, are associated with nature and life. It's this sort of green that you can see if you go to a local park or wildlife preserve, and experts encourage exposure to. A literature review suggests that "exposure to green, relative to other colors, slowed down heart rate in walking and increased perceived exertion" (Briki & Majed, 2019). This means that you are more likely to be productive in an environment where you are surrounded by a natural color, such as green.

Another environmental change you could make is to minimize distractions. Turn off any sources of unwanted noise, such as televisions, computer games, cellphones, and other electronic devices. Close a window if the noises of the outside world are becoming too much for you. We live in a noisy world, full of things to occupy our time and attention, and it's the greatest act of rebellion to reclaim our right to peace and quiet.

We have discussed nutrition and its relation to hormone balance, although we have not fully discussed how to implement it. If you want to change your diet and eat a little healthier, simply try and have healthy food around the house. Buy fruits and vegetables you know you like and that you know you will eat. Avoid listening to social media "wellness influencers" who are out to demonize the foods you like, and who want to push restrictive diet patterns as "the ultimate diet for optimal health." The "optimal diet" is the diet that you can follow for the rest of your life, and it might mean making a few smart swaps. For example:

- Using honey in place of refined sugar

- Swapping to water or decaffeinated drinks in the morning instead of coffee

- Drinking fizzy water instead of the full sugar variety

- Aiming to eat at least three servings of vegetables per day

- Eating more lean meats like turkey and chicken

- Cutting back on processed foods, such as potato chips and candy, and instead opting for rice cakes, a handful of nuts, or fruit as a replacement

- Using reduced sodium salt and other seasonings when cooking

There's nothing wrong with enjoying candy, chocolate, potato chips, or whatever your favorite snack is. However, when we come to rely on these things and we eat them every single day, they become a core part of our diet, and we begin to feel the consequences. Potato chips are a huge contributor to high sodium intake. While it's fine to enjoy them, opt for the low-sodium version, choose a smaller package if it's available, or cut down on your overall potato chip intake. This is the same for chocolate. Most chocolate in the United States does not contain cocoa powder, a key ingredient in chocolate. It's mostly cocoa fat and sugar, which are addictive and high in calories. Opt for high-quality dark chocolate (at least 70% cocoa) or milk chocolate with a high cocoa percentage instead.

If you don't want to take supplements, another thing to try is to increase your intake of dark, leafy green vegetables and lean red meats. These foods will give you most of your dietary iron, magnesium, and B12 intake for the day. If you "eat the rainbow" anyway, there is a good chance you are getting everything you need in your diet, and you don't need to take supplements. Speak with a registered dietitian if you want to learn more about the best way to nourish your body to prevent and manage hormonal imbalances.

Stress Management Strategies

Stress management is a skill that everyone needs. We all think we're great at managing our stress, when in fact we're not as good as we could be. We've all done that workplace seminar where we learn about communication, using a stress ball, and taking deep breaths, but that information can be forgotten almost as quickly as we learn it. This is why habit formation is so critical to hormone balance: Instead of actually utilizing the skills we learn, we toss them to the side and carry on with our lives. That's because the skills we learn in the workplace are only workable in the workplace. We need *lifestyle* stress management skills in order to form healthy habits.

The secret? Find the cause of your stress. Grab the stress ball, but don't rely on it. Acute stress is fine as it's short-term and disappears after a while. However, chronic stress is where problems begin to manifest. Maintaining stress management is how we avoid worse problems being brought about by chronic stress. You can do this, as mentioned, by *getting to the root of what is stressing you out*. Journaling every day can present recurring themes in your life and may even hit you with an "Aha!" moment of why you are stressed. Journaling also serves as a sort of "ranting" mechanism, while letting you air out your frustrations in a healthy way.

I recommend cutting back on your caffeine intake. I love a cup of coffee just as much as the next person, but caffeine is a stimulant, and it can increase your heart rate. This tells the body that it's in danger, and the parasympathetic nervous system begins releasing cortisol and adrenaline in order to prepare you for it. The body does not know that you're drinking coffee as a means of your "wake up" routine, it just knows that it's suddenly stimulated and you might need to fight off a bear, so that's what it's preparing you for. The daily recommended intake of caffeine is 400 mg. A large latte from Starbucks has around 150 mg of caffeine, so it only takes three large lattes to put you over the limit. Around 8 oz of black coffee has 100 mg of caffeine, making it a little safer. Depending on how much you've had, caffeine can linger for up to six hours. Switch to decaf a few hours before going to bed, after eating lunch, and over the next few weeks, making note of how you feel and try to build this habit.

Health Screenings: A Reminder

We have covered the importance of health screenings in-depth, so take this short section as a reminder that going to the doctor does not need to be a bad experience. Your doctor is trained to become an expert in their field, and they are under a series of pressures and restrictions that greatly affect their ability to provide the care they want to give. You are also not their only patient; they have dozens of people they need to see every day, so their time and attention are limited. This is why you should ask for a longer appointment if needed, and go in with a list of pre-prepared questions and any knowledge you can gather about your family's history of hormonal conditions. Well-informed self-diagnosis can be helpful, and you can use this to your advantage. However, if you go into the doctor's office saying, "I related to a video I saw on TikTok," you will not be taken as seriously as if you say, "This hormonal condition runs in my family; I'm concerned I might be at risk for it, and I've looked into the research and would like to take it further."

Hormonal imbalances and certain conditions have very strict diagnostic criteria, which can greatly affect the way we handle ourselves, and the medical treatment we receive. If you live in the United States, these tests can be difficult and expensive to come by. That's why, before you go to the doctor, you need to look through your insurance policy to find out exactly what it covers and how much you need to pay before insurance will cover it. It is also helpful to get confirmation of that in writing. You want to be able to challenge any discrepancies or denials that crop up because you want the best case you can possibly build.

It's also worth noting that in many cases, your doctor can only provide the care that someone high above them has approved. This is why you need to be the one to make the case. You're not just trying to convince your doctor, but you're trying to cut through the red tape and get the care you know you deserve.

Conclusion

The body needs stress to some degree in order to keep things running efficiently. Remember how the body loves homeostasis? Well, it needs a reason to keep working toward it, and stress is what gives it that motivation. However, if you are suffering from severe and chronic bouts of stress for extended periods of time, it can begin to have consequences. These consequences tend to wreak havoc on your hormones, and this can damage vital systems in the body. The central nervous system might start to malfunction if you are in a constant state of fight-or-flight, and your immune system will stop working.

Lifestyle changes are key to maintaining a healthy hormone balance. This is because the body does require stimulation and some stress, but it also requires adequate rest and relaxation. This will provide your body with the energy it requires to function. There are many things you can do to allow your body to recover and heal from bouts of stress. You can delegate work duties to others instead of taking on everything yourself. You can also use your sick days and paid time off. Make time for yourself, and if that means carving out half an hour a day to do some breathing exercises or simply enjoy a cup of tea, do it.

Other lifestyle changes include reducing your caffeine and alcohol consumption. The things we put into our bodies greatly affect what happens *inside* of us, and it's important that we understand that. While it's okay to enjoy these things once in a while with little consequence, making a habit of it will turn it into something we rely on, and this can cause hormonal imbalances.

Chapter 12:

Resources and Communities

This chapter will be less about how to maintain your hormone balance, and more of a valuable resource hub. I have found an abundance of trusted and accessible tools for those seeking to achieve optimal hormonal health. There are a variety of online and offline resources, including informative websites, educational books, podcasts, support groups, and expert consultations. I cannot impress the importance of community support enough. Shared experiences in managing women's hormonal health can make or break a person's ability to trust themselves. There are various social networks and community platforms where women can discuss, learn, and empower each other, and I am here to steer you in that direction.

Online Resources

Websites and Forums

North American Menopause Society (NAMS)

Let's Talk Menopause

Office on Women's Health

World Health Organization

- Menopause
- PCOS

Patients Like Me

Ask Early Menopause

Blogs and Articles

Medical News Today: "What to Know About Hormonal Imbalances"

Healthline: "Everything You Should Know About Hormonal Imbalance"

AIA: "Eight Signs of Hormonal Imbalance That Need Checking"

Research Journal of Life Sciences, Bioinformatics, Pharmaceutical and Chemical Sciences: "Hormone Imbalance—A Cause for Concern in Women"

Podcasts

The No Sugarcoating Podcast

Healthy Hormones for Women

The 4 Phase Cycle Podcast

You and Your Hormones

The Dr. Louise Newson Podcast

Books

Finally, below is a short list of books that I have found helpful in understanding my own hormone health:

- *Hormones, Health, and Human Potential* by Dr. Nicky Keay
- *When You're Ready, This Is How You Heal* by Brianna Wiest
- *The Hormone Balance Bible* by Shawn Tassone
- *Natural Solutions to PCOS* by Marilyn Glenville
- *Young Forever* by Dr. Mark Hyman

Conclusion

Balancing our hormones is more complicated than we think. While it can be as simple as, "I'm hungry, so my blood sugar is low," it can be as complicated as "certain gene mutations influence the metabolism of different hormones."

The body has hormones for everything, and those hormones are regulated by various systems throughout the body. Your circadian rhythms, specifically your sleep/wake cycle, play a role in your hormonal balance. When it gets dark outside, you might start to feel sleepy because melatonin is being secreted. When you drink coffee to wake up, it's because the intake of caffeine has stimulated the release of adrenaline and cortisol. Other hormones include ghrelin and leptin, which regulate hunger, and the sex hormones, estrogen and progesterone.

Estrogen is an umbrella term for different hormones that play different roles in puberty, development, and fertility. While it is considered the primary female hormone, it is not the only sex hormone women possess. Women also have testosterone and other androgens, or "male hormones." These androgens play key roles in sex drive, hair growth, and muscle development.

A woman will go through many hormonal stages throughout her life. Throughout puberty, the pituitary gland will release human growth hormone, her ovaries will release estrogen and progesterone, and her body will take on the characteristics of a woman—broad hips, breasts, and menstruation. Menstruation is the second most significant hormonal change, as it is the cycle that governs fertility. Later in life, a woman will experience perimenopause and finally, menopause which are both characterized by fluctuations and eventual ceasing of the female sex hormones.

However, there are many different hormonal conditions that exist outside of the hormonal stages. The most common among women are Hashimoto's disease, polycystic ovary syndrome, and type 2 diabetes. The signs and symptoms of these conditions are not unique and can be mistaken or crossed over with other conditions. This is what prompts many women to self-diagnose or become engrossed in literature surrounding specific conditions.

Although a well-informed self-diagnosis can be useful, it can also be detrimental. Most conditions, such as Hashimoto's disease and polycystic ovary syndrome, have specific diagnostic criteria that help to inform the course of treatment. A woman who diagnoses herself with diabetes may find herself on a dangerous fasting regimen that will damage her hormone balance even more. In going about self-diagnosis, you need to be aware of your family's history and whether or not these conditions are already present. However, it is always best to seek medical advice.

Seeking medical advice does not need to be scary. I understand why some women might want to avoid going to the doctor. Our hormonal health is often looked at by society as an inconvenience to others. Unfortunately, it's also a *vital* part of our health, which is why advocating for ourselves is necessary.

There are plenty of factors that affect hormonal health. The body is a huge fan of homeostasis, and it will fight for homeostasis. It's also important to remember that not all chemicals are bad because everything is a chemical. Water is a chemical. Your blood is a chemical. Manufactured chemicals that mimic certain hormones, on the other hand, *can* be a problem because they interrupt homeostasis. This is why it's so important to wear personal protective equipment when using them. Other factors include environmental pollution, local climate, and your diet and lifestyle.

In the same sense that there are many things that can cause your hormones to go out of balance, there are plenty of things you can do to get them back into balance. These include going to the doctor and receiving a diagnosis if you suspect that you have a hormonal imbalance disorder. Type 2 diabetes, for example, can be treated with exogenous insulin. You can also increase your physical activity to better regulate your adrenaline and cortisol levels, cut back on your caffeine intake, and give your body the nourishment it needs to thrive. Regular yoga and breathwork can also help to soothe the nervous system, which will release endorphins and help you relax.

The body can withstand a lot of things. It's a machine—a master recycler—and it knows what it needs.

Your hormonal health is so important, and you should think of it as such. In light of this, you should endeavor to learn as much about it as you possibly can. Instead of accepting your fate and allowing your body to break down during menopause or as a result of a clinically diagnosed condition, take action and learn about your body. Learn how to keep it healthy and balanced. This doesn't just apply to hormonal conditions like PCOS or Hashimoto's, but it applies to women who are, otherwise, healthy.

Now that you are armed with the knowledge you need to restore and regulate your own hormone levels and how to advocate for yourself, I wish you all the best. You got this! Remember to regulate your sleep cycle, increase the nutritional value of your diet, and get moving. Your body is a temple, honor it as such.

Embark on Your Hormone-Balancing Journey Here!

As you conclude your journey through "Balance Restored," we extend our heartfelt gratitude for accompanying us on this transformative path. In celebration of your commitment to reclaiming your hormone health, we are thrilled to present you with an exclusive gift – "Balanced Bites."

"Balanced Bites" is a powerful eBook meticulously crafted to complement your quest for hormonal harmony. Within its virtual embrace, you will discover a concise overview of essential hormone-supporting nutrients, a must-have shopping list for nurturing hormonal balance, and an array of delectable hormone-balancing recipes spanning breakfast, lunch, dinner, snacks, and desserts, each accompanied by its nutritional breakdown.

To access your special gift, simply scan the QR code below and follow the straightforward steps. Embrace this invaluable resource and let it serve as a guiding light illuminating your path toward holistic well-being.

As you set forth on your extraordinary voyage toward understanding and embracing the exquisite harmony of hormone balance, we invite you to share your reflections on

"Balance Restored." If the insights and knowledge within its pages have inspired you, kindly consider leaving a review, empowering others to embark on this profound journey.

With warmest wishes for abundant health and joy.

Olivia Rivers

References

Abel, A. N., Lloyd, L. K., & Williams, J. S. (2013, March 20). *The effects of regular yoga practice on pulmonary function in healthy individuals: A literature review.* The Journal of Alternative and Complementary Medicine, *19*(3), 185–190. https://doi.org/10.1089/acm.2011.0516

Acidosis: MedlinePlus medical encyclopedia. (2021). MedlinePlus. https://medlineplus.gov/ency/article/001181.htm

Androgen deficiency in women. (2022, November 22). Better Health. https://www.betterhealth.vic.gov.au/health/conditions andtreatments/androgen-deficiency-in-women#symptoms-of-androgen-deficiency

Baird, P. A., Anderson, T. W., Newcombe, H. B., & Lowry, R. B. (1988, May). *Genetic disorders in children and young adults: A population study.* National Library of Medicine, 42(5), 677–693. https://www.ncbi.nlm.nih.gov/pmc/articles/PMC1715177/

Bessell, E., Maunder, A., Lauche, R., Adams, J., Sainsbury, A., & Fuller, N. R. (2021, May 11). *Efficacy of dietary supplements containing isolated organic compounds for weight loss: A systematic review and meta-analysis of randomised placebo-controlled trials.* International Journal of Obesity, *45*(8), 1631–1643. https://doi.org/10.1038/s41366-021-00839-w

Bhimwal, T., Priyadarshani, P., & Priyadarshani, A. (2023). *Understanding polycystic ovary syndrome in light of associated key genes*. Egyptian Journal of Medical Human Genetics, 24(1). https://doi.org/10.1186/s43042-023-00418-w

Bova, T. L., Chiavaccini, L., Cline, G. F., Hart, C. G., Matheny, K., Muth, A. M., Voelz, B. E., Kesler, D., & Memili, E. (2014). *Environmental stressors influencing hormones and systems physiology in cattle*. Reproductive Biology and Endocrinology, 12, 58. https://doi.org/10.1186/1477-7827-12-58

Boyle, N.B., Lawton, C., & Dye, L. (2017, April 26). *The effects of magnesium supplementation on subjective anxiety and stress—a systematic review*. Nutrients, 9(5), 429. https://doi.org/10.3390/nu9050429

Briki, W., & Majed, L. (2019, February 12). *Adaptive effects of seeing green environment on psychophysiological parameters when walking or running*. Frontiers in Psychology, 10(252). https://doi.org/10.3389/fpsyg.2019.00252

Buck-Flamingo, A. (2023, August 15). *Studies show what America's sickest days are*. TheHRDirector. https://www.thehrdirector.com/features/absence-management/studies-show-americas-sickest-days/

Chen, L., Deng, H., Cui, H., Fang, J., Zuo, Z., Deng, J., Li, Y., Wang, X., & Zhao, L. (2018). *Inflammatory responses and inflammation-associated diseases in organs*. Oncotarget, 9(6), 7204–7218. https://doi.org/10.18632/oncotarget.23208

Circadian rhythms. (2023, August 15). National Institute of General Medical Sciences. https://nigms.nih.gov/education/fact-sheets/Pages/Circadian-Rhythms.aspx

Clark, T. D., Reichelt, A. C., Ghosh-Swaby, O., Simpson, S. J., & Crean, A. J. (2022, April). *Nutrition, anxiety and* hormones. *Why sex differences matter in the link between obesity and behavior.* Physiology & Behavior, 247, 113713. https://doi.org/10.1016/j.physbeh.2022.113713

Clear, J. (2018). *Atomic habits.* Penguin Publishing Group.

Cole, J. B., & Florez, J. C. (2020). *Genetics of diabetes mellitus and diabetes complications.* Nature Reviews. Nephrology, 16(7). https://doi.org/10.1038/s41581-020-0278-5

Copeland, J. L., Consitt, L. A., & Tremblay, M. S. (2002, April 1). *Hormonal responses to endurance and resistance exercise in females aged 19-69 years.* The Journals of Gerontology Series A: Gerontological Society of America. 57(4), B158–B165.
https://doi.org/10.1093/gerona/57.4.b158

Lee, D. (2020, April 15). *Could hormone replacement therapy boost your immune system?* Open Access Government. https://www.openaccessgovernment.org/hormone-replacement-therapy-boost-your-immune-system/85516/

Lysebeth, André Van. (2007). *Pranayama: The energetics of breath: The yoga of breathing.* Harmony.

Cropley, M., Banks, A. P., & Boyle, J. (2015, October 27). *The effects of rhodiola rosea L. extract on anxiety, stress, cognition and other mood symptoms.* Phytotherapy Research: PTR, 29(12), 1934–1939. https://doi.org/10.1002/ptr.5486

Dashti, H. S., Scheer, F. A., Jacques, P. F., Lamon-Fava, S., & Ordovás, J. M. (2015, November). *Short sleep duration and dietary intake: Epidemiologic evidence, mechanisms, and health implications.* Advances in Nutrition, 6(6), 648–659. https://doi.org/10.3945/an.115.008623

De Leo, V., Musacchio, M. C., Cappelli, V., Massaro, M. G., Morgante, G., & Petraglia, F. (2016). *Genetic, hormonal and metabolic aspects of PCOS: An update.* Reproductive Biology and Endocrinology, 14(1). https://doi.org/10.1186/s12958-016-0173-x

Desai, R., Tailor, A., & Bhatt, T. (2015, May). *Effects of yoga on brain waves and structural activation: A review.* Complementary Therapies in Clinical Practice, 21(2), 112–118. https://doi.org/10.1016/j.ctcp.2015.02.002

Donovitz, G. S. (2022, July 22). *A personal prospective on testosterone therapy in women—what we know in 2022.* Journal of Personalized Medicine, 12(8), 1194. https://doi.org/10.3390/jpm12081194

Eight signs of hormonal imbalance that need checking. (2023, April 27). AIA. https://www.aia.com/en/health-wellness/healthy-living/healthy-body/Hormonal-imbalance-in-women

Elflein, J. (2023, September 21). *Number of sick days taken in the past 12 months from work or school/university among adults in the U.S. from 2022 to 2023.* Statista. https://www.statista.com/forecasts/1260743/number-of-sick-days-taken-from-work-or-school-among-us-adults

Endocrine-disrupting chemicals (EDCs) (2022, January 24) Endocrine Society. https://www.endocrine.org/patient-engagement/endocrine-library/edcs

Endocrine: Genetic syndromes. (n.d.). Baylor College of Medicine. https://www.bcm.edu/healthcare/specialties/endocrinology/endocrinology-diabetes-and-metabolism/adrenal-disorders/endocrine-genetic-syndromes

Ennour-Idrissi, K., Maunsell, E., & Diorio, C. (2015). *Effect of physical activity on sex hormones in women: A systematic review and meta-analysis of randomized controlled trials.* Breast Cancer Research, 17(1). https://doi.org/10.1186/s13058-015-0647-3

Escobar, G. J., & Dellinger, R. P. (2016, November). *Early detection, prevention, and mitigation of critical illness outside intensive care settings.* Journal of Hospital Medicine, 11, S5–S10. https://doi.org/10.1002/jhm.2653

Foresta, C., Zuccarello, D., Garolla, A., & Ferlin, A. (2008, August 1). *Role of hormones, genes, and environment in human cryptorchidism.* Endocrine Reviews, 29(5), 560–580. https://doi.org/10.1210/er.2007-0042

Francina, S. (2015, October 27). *Yoga and the wisdom of menopause: A guide to physical, emotional, and spiritual health at midlife and beyond.* Health Communications.

Frequency of fatigue-related crashes. (n.d.). European Commission. https://road-safety.transport.ec.europa.eu/european-road-safety-observatory/statistics-and-analysis-archive/fatigue/frequency-fatigue-related-crashes_en

From fatigue to flow: How iron can help during your period. (2023, April 20). Your Wellness Collective. https://yourwellnesscollective.ie/en-gb/blogs/your-wellness-collective-blog/from-fatigue-to-flow-how-iron-can-help-you-during-their-period

Fruhwürth, S., Vogel, H., Schürmann, A., & Williams, K. J. (2018). *Novel insights into how overnutrition disrupts the hypothalamic actions of leptin.* Frontiers in Endocrinology, 9. https://doi.org/10.3389/fendo.2018.00089

Furhad, S., & Bokhari, A. A. (2023, July 19). *Herbal supplements*. StatPearls Publishing. https://www.ncbi.nlm.nih.gov/books/NBK536964/

Gao, Q., & Horvath, T. L. (2008). *Cross-talk between estrogen and leptin signaling in the hypothalamus*. American Journal of Physiology-Endocrinology and Metabolism, 294(5), E817–E826. https://doi.org/10.1152/ajpendo.00733.2007

Genetic syndromes. (n.d.). UCLA Health. https://www.uclahealth.org/medical-services/surgery/endocrine-surgery/conditions-treated/genetic-syndromes

Gharahdaghi, N., Phillips, B. E., Szewczyk, N. J., Smith, K., Wilkinson, D. J., & Atherton, P. J. (2021, January 15). *Links between testosterone, oestrogen, and the growth hormone/insulin-like growth factor axis and resistance exercise muscle adaptations*. Frontiers in Physiology, 11. https://doi.org/10.3389/fphys.2020.621226

Glenville, M. (2012). *Natural solutions to PCOS: How to eliminate your symptoms and boost your fertility*. Macmillan.

Gottlieb, D. J., Ellenbogen, J. M., Bianchi, M. T., & Czeisler, C. A. (2018, March 20). *Sleep deficiency and motor vehicle crash risk in the general population: A prospective cohort study*. BMC Medicine, 16(1). https://doi.org/10.1186/s12916-018-1025-7

Hackney, A. C. (2017). *Sex hormones, exercise and women: Scientific and clinical aspects*. Springer.

Hackney, A. C., & Lane, A. R. (2015). *Chapter twelve - exercise and the regulation of endocrine hormones* (C. Bouchard, Ed.). ScienceDirect; Academic Press.

https://www.sciencedirect.com/science/article/abs/pii/S1877117315001337

Hayden, A. (2022). *Findings on HRT since the women's health initiative*. Women's Health Network. https://www.womenshealthnetwork.com/hrt/womens-health-initiative-new-findings/

Helm, J. S., Nishioka, M., Brody, J. G., Rudel, R. A., & Dodson, R. E. (2018, August). *Measurement of endocrine disrupting and asthma-associated chemicals in hair products used by black women*. Environmental Research, 165, 448–458. https://doi.org/10.1016/j.envres.2018.03.030

Herrera, A. Y., Nielsen, S. E., & Mather, M. (2016, June). *Stress-induced increases in progesterone and cortisol in naturally cycling women*. Neurobiology of Stress, 3, 96–104. https://doi.org/10.1016/j.ynstr.2016.02.006

Hieter, P., Andrews, B., Fowler, D. M., & Bellen, H. (2023, August). *Highlighting rare disease research with a genetics and series on genetic models of rare diseases*. Genetics, 224(4). https://doi.org/10.1093/genetics/iyad121

Hormones: The inside story - podcast. (n.d.). You and Your Hormones. https://www.yourhormones.info/resources/digital-library/podcasts/

How does food affect your hormones? (n.d.). The Marion Gluck Clinic. https://www.mariongluckclinic.com/blog/how-does-food-affect-your-hormones.html

How to talk to your GP about menopause. (n.d.). University of Glasgow. https://www.gla.ac.uk/myglasgow/humanresources/all/health/menopause/guidance-howtotalktoyourgpaboutmenopause/

Huizen.J., *What to know about hormonal imbalance*s. (2023, October 23). Medical News Today. https://www.medicalnewstoday.com/articles/321486

Hyman, M. (2023). *Young Forever.* Little, Brown Spark.

Is Hashimoto's disease hereditary? (2022, September 17). HealthMatch. https://healthmatch.io/hashimotos-disease/is-hashimotos-disease-hereditary#hashimoto-s-disease-symptoms

Iyengar, B. K. S. (2013). *Light on pranayama: The definitive guide to the art of breathing.* Harper Collins.

James, M. (2022, November 27). *Talking to your doctor about hormone therapy.* Women's Health Network. https://www.womenshealthnetwork.com/hrt/hormone-therapy-talking-to-your-doctor/

Jia, J., Cameron, N. A., & Linder, J. A. (2022, June 21). *Multivitamins and Supplements—Benign Prevention or Potentially Harmful Distraction?* JAMA, 327(23), 2294. https://doi.org/10.1001/jama.2022.9167

Keay, N. (2022). *Hormones, health and human potential: A guide to understanding your hormones to optimize your health & performance.* Sequoia Books.

Khan, M. J., Ullah, A., & Basit, S. (2019, December 24). *Genetic basis of polycystic ovary syndrome (PCOS): Current perspectives.* The Application of Clinical Genetics, Volume 12(12), 249–260. https://doi.org/10.2147/tacg.s200341

Kim, T. W., Jeong, J.-H., & Hong, S.-C. (2015). *The impact of sleep and circadian disturbance on hormones and metabolism.* International Journal of Endocrinology, 2015(591729), 1–9. https://doi.org/10.1155/2015/591729

Kubala, J., & Van De Walle, G. (2023, March 31). *7 science-backed health benefits of rhodiola rosea.* Healthline. https://www.healthline.com/nutrition/rhodiola-rosea

Lang, A. (2023, August 7). *10 natural ways to balance your hormones.* Healthline Media. https://www.healthline.com/nutrition/balance-hormones

Leal, D. (2020). *10 superfoods to eat daily for optimal health.* Verywell Fit. https://www.verywellfit.com/eat-a-wide-variety-of-superfoods-3121399

Lee, I., & Ji, K. (2022). *Identification of combinations of endocrine disrupting chemicals in household chemical products that require mixture toxicity testing.* Ecotoxicology and Environmental Safety, 240, 113677. https://doi.org/10.1016/j.ecoenv.2022.113677

Lee, J. R., & Hopkins, V. (2006). *Dr. John Lee's Hormone Balance Made Simple: The essential how-to guide to symptoms, dosage, timing, and more.* Health & Fitness.

Lee, S. R., Choi, W.-Y., Heo, J. H., Huh, J., Kim, G., Lee, K.-P., Kwun, H.-J., Shin, H.-J., Baek, I.-J., & Hong, E.-J. (2020, October 1). *Progesterone increases blood glucose via hepatic progesterone receptor membrane component 1 under limited or impaired action of insulin.* Scientific Reports, 10(1), 16316. https://doi.org/10.1038/s41598-020-73330-7

Let's talk menopause (n.d.). https://www.letstalkmenopause.org/

Maghnie, M., Loche, S., Cappa, M., Ghizzoni, L., & Lorini. R. (2013). *Hormone resistance and hypersensitivity: From genetics to clinical management.* Karger.

Martín-Pozo, L., Gómez-Regalado, M. del C., Moscoso-Ruiz, I., & Zafra-Gómez, A. (2021, November 1). *Analytical methods for the determination of endocrine disrupting chemicals in cosmetics and personal care products: A review.* Talanta, 234, 122642. https://doi.org/10.1016/j.talanta.2021.122642

Menopause (2022, October 17) World Health Organization. https://www.who.int/news-room/fact-sheets/detail/menopause

Menstrual cycle (n.d.) Better Health Channel. https://www.betterhealth.vic.gov.au/health/conditions andtreatments/menstrual-cycle

Micronutrients. (n.d.). World Health Organization. https://www.who.int/health-topics/micronutrients#tab=tab_1

Mintz, J., Mirza, J., Young, E., & Bauckman, K. (2020, December 8). *Iron therapeutics in women's health: Past, present, and future.* Pharmaceuticals, 13(12), 449. https://doi.org/10.3390/ph13120449

Miraglia, C., Moccia, F., Russo, M., Scida, S., Franceschi, M., Crafa, P., Franzoni, L., Nouvenne, A., Meschi, T., Leandro, G., De' Angelis, G. L., & Di Mario, F. (2018). *Non-invasive method for the assessment of gastric acid secretion.* Acta Biomedia: Atenei Parmensis, 89(8-S), 53–57. https://doi.org/10.23750/abm.v89i8-S.7986

Munisamy, N., & Tringham, J. (2021). *Is Aloe vera always beneficial?* Endocrine Abstracts. https://doi.org/10.1530/endoabs.77.lb29

North American Menopause Society (NAMS) Promoting women's health at midlife and beyond. (n.d.). https://www.menopause.org/

Nowell, C. (2023, June 23). *Flamin' hot addictions: Why is America so hooked on ultra-processed foods?* The Guardian. https://www.theguardian.com/environment/2023/jun/23/processed-foods-american-addiction

O'Rourke, J. A., Ravichandran, C., Howe, Y. J., Mullett, J. E., Keary, C. J., Golas, S. B., Hureau, A. R., McCormick, M., Chung, J., Rose, N. R., & McDougle, C. J. (2019, May 29). *Accuracy of self-reported history of autoimmune disease: A pilot study.* PLOS ONE, 14(5), e0216526. https://doi.org/10.1371/journal.pone.0216526

Parazzini, F., Di Martino, M., & Pellegrino, P. (2017, February 1). *Magnesium in the gynecological practice: A literature review.* Magnesium Research, 30(1), 1–7. https://doi.org/10.1684/mrh.2017.0419

Pashayan, N., Antoniou, A. C., Ivanus, U., Esserman, L. J., Easton, D. F., French, D., Sroczynski, G., Hall, P., Cuzick, J., Evans, D. G., Simard, J., Garcia-Closas, M., Schmutzler, R., Wegwarth, O., Pharoah, P., Moorthie, S., De Montgolfier, S., Baron, C., Herceg, Z., & Turnbull, C. (2020, June 18). *Personalized early detection and prevention of breast cancer: ENVISION consensus statement.* Nature Reviews Clinical Oncology. https://doi.org/10.1038/s41571-020-0388-9

Polycystic ovary syndrome. (2023, June 28). World Health Organization. https://www.who.int/news-room/fact-sheets/detail/polycystic-ovary-syndrome

Prasad, D., Wollenhaupt-Aguiar, B., Kidd, K. N., de Azevedo Cardoso, T., & Frey, B. N. (2021, December 16). *Suicidal risk in women with premenstrual syndrome and premenstrual dysphoric disorder: A systematic review and meta-analysis.* Journal of Women's Health, 30(12). https://doi.org/10.1089/jwh.2021.0185

Premenstrual dysphoric disorder PMDD. (n.d.). Mind. https://www.mind.org.uk/information-support/types-of-mental-health-problems/premenstrual-dysphoric-disorder-pmdd/about-pmdd/

Razzaque, M. (2018). *Magnesium: Are we consuming enough?* Nutrients, 10(12), 1863. https://doi.org/10.3390/nu10121863

Roop, J.K. (2018). *Hormone Imbalance - A cause for concern in women.* Research Journal of Life Sciences, Bioinformatics, Pharmaceutical, and Chemical Sciences, https://doi.org/10.26479/2018.0402.18

Salve, J., Pate, S., Debnath, K., & Langade, D. (2019, December 25). *Adaptogenic and Anxiolytic Effects of Ashwagandha Root Extract in Healthy Adults: A Double-blind, Randomized, Placebo-controlled Clinical Study.* Cureus, 11(12). https://doi.org/10.7759/cureus.6466

Sam, S. (2007). *Obesity and polycystic ovary syndrome.* Obesity Management, 3(2), 69–73. https://doi.org/10.1089/obe.2007.0019

Sardashti, S. & Abadi, Tahere & Abadi, Shoaib & Raznahan, Rasool. (2020). *Investigation the effect of oral Aloe Vera gel pills supplementation on the intensity of primary menstrual pain (Dysmenorrhea).* Balneo Research Journal. 11. 120-124. 10.12680/balneo.2020.326.

Spilling the beans: How much caffeine is too much? (n.d.). U.S. Food & Drug Administration. https://www.fda.gov/consumers/consumer-updates/spilling-beans-how-much-caffeine-too-much

Starr, J. (2011). *The effect of melatonin on the ovaries.* The Science Journal of the Lander College of Arts and Sciences, 5.

https://touroscholar.touro.edu/cgi/viewcontent.cgi?article=1138&context=sjlcas

Sulanc, E. (2021, November). *Is thyroid cancer really more common in women than men?* American Thyroid Association. https://www.thyroid.org/patient-thyroid-information/ct-for-patients/november-2021/vol-14-issue-11-p-11-12/

Tabackman, L. (2023, April 7). *Is type 2 diabetes genetic?* Healthline. https://www.healthline.com/health/type-2-diabetes/genetics#responsible-genes

Tassone, S. (2021). *The Hormone Balance Bible.* HarperCollins.

10 best hormone balancing podcasts. (2023, November 30). FeedSpot for Podcasters. https://podcasts.feedspot.com/hormone_balancing_podcasts/

Travers, C. (2023). *Decoding hormone imbalances in women.* The Well by Northwell. https://thewell.northwell.edu/womens-health/hormone-imbalance-symptoms

Turske, C. (2011). *Hormone balance through yoga: A pocket guide for women over 40.* Hunter House.

Urban, M. (1999). *Early observations of genetic diseases.* The Lancet, 354, SIV21. https://doi.org/10.1016/s0140-6736(99)90364-1

Vallée, A., Ceccaldi, P-F., Carbonnel, M., Anis Féki, & Ayoubi, J.-M. (2023, October 9). *Pollution and endometriosis: A deep dive into the environmental impacts on women's health.* Bjog: An International Journal of Obstetrics and Gynaecology. https://doi.org/10.1111/1471-0528.17687

Wadden, T. A., Mason, G., Foster, G. D., Stunkard, A. J., & Prange, A. J. (1990). *Effects of a very low calorie diet on weight, thyroid hormones and mood.* International Journal of Obesity, 14(3), 249–258. https://pubmed.ncbi.nlm.nih.gov/2341229/

What are sleep deprivation and deficiency? (2022, March 24). National Heart, Lung, and Blood Institute. https://www.nhlbi.nih.gov/health/sleep-deprivation

What do I need to tell the doctor? (n.d.) National Institute on Aging. https://www.nia.nih.gov/health/what-do-i-need-tell-doctor

Willemsen, G., Ward, K. J., Bell, C. G., Christensen, K., Bowden, J., Dalgård, C., Harris, J. R., Kaprio, J., Lyle, R., Magnusson, P. K. E., Mather, K. A., Ordoñana, J. R., Perez-Riquelme, F., Pedersen, N. L., Pietiläinen, K. H., Sachdev, P. S., Boomsma, D. I., & Spector, T. (2015, December 18). *The concordance and heritability of type 2 diabetes in 34,166 twin pairs from international twin registers: The discordant twin (DISCOTWIN) consortium.* Twin Research and Human Genetics, 18(6), 762–771. https://doi.org/10.1017/thg.2015.83

Woodward, A., Klonizakis, M., & Broom, D. (2020, April 28). *Exercise and Polycystic Ovary Syndrome.* Physical Exercise for Human Health, 1228, 123–136. https://doi.org/10.1007/978-981-15-1792-1_8

Ye, L., & Ning, G. (2015, July 7). *The molecular classification of hereditary endocrine diseases.* Endocrine, 50(3), 575–579. https://doi.org/10.1007/s12020-015-0674-y

Yeung, E. H., Zhang, C., Mumford, S. L., Ye, A., Trevisan, M., Chen, L., Browne, R. W., Wactawski-Wende, J., & Schisterman, E. F. (2010, December 1). *Longitudinal study of insulin resistance and sex hormones over the menstrual cycle: The biocycle study*. The Journal of Clinical Endocrinology & Metabolism, 95(12), 5435–5442. https://doi.org/10.1210/jc.2010-0702

Yu, M., Feng, R., Sun, X., Wang, H., Wang, H., Sang, Q., Jin, L., He, L., & Wang, L. (2014, March 9). *Polymorphisms of pentanucleotide repeats (tttta)n in the promoter of CYP11A1 and their relationships to polycystic ovary syndrome (PCOS) risk: A meta-analysis*. Molecular Biology Reports, 41(7), 4435–4445. https://doi.org/10.1007/s11033-014-3314-3

Zhang, Y., Xun, P., Wang, R., Mao, L., & He, K. (2017). *Can magnesium enhance exercise performance?* Nutrients, 9(9), 946. https://doi.org/10.3390/nu9090946

Printed in Great Britain
by Amazon